American Medical Associa
Physicians dedicated to the health of America

The
Medical
Marriage

Sustaining Healthy Relationships for Physicians and Their Families

Wayne M. Sotile, Ph.D.
Mary O. Sotile, M.A.

Foreword by Michael Myers, M.D.

Revised Edition

Additional copies may be ordered from:
Order Department OP209200
ISBN 1-57947-075-0
American Medical Association
For order information, call toll-free 800 621-8335.

BP37:03-P-061:2/03

Dedication

To the thousands of physicians and their loved ones who have privileged us with private glimpses into the inner workings of their homes and hearts. We admire and appreciate your courage; you are the heroes.

Foreword

When I graduated from medical school in 1966, I remember only one professor who made any reference to our lives outside of medicine. His words were, "Marry a strong woman, because she will have to do everything at home—your first duty must be to medicine."

Interesting statement, given that there were seven women in our class (and possibly one or more students who were not heterosexual). Although we have evolved leaps and bounds since the mid-60s, many medical students and residents today are still made to feel that their marriages (or other committed relationships) must take a secondary position behind their medical work.

Further, with some notable exceptions, attendings and mentors do not "teach" balance or act as role models. Many are embarrassed about strain at home and, feeling overworked and helpless, don't know what to do about it. To quote a patient of mine, a respected academic physician with three children: "I'm ashamed of my personal life. I'm on a treadmill that I can't get off of. I hardly see my wife and kids. They have no interest in me and what I do. Is this a lifestyle that I want to teach my residents and fellows?"

It is no secret that marriages of physicians can be tough going. Given the personality characteristics of individuals who choose medicine as a career, the fact that many of these individuals have nuclear conflicts with intimacy, the delayed maturity associated with a long course of study, and the overall seriousness of the work (and the awesome responsibility to patients), it is difficult for some physicians to give love unwaveringly to their families—and to feel loved in return.

Classically, and somewhat paradoxically, physicians do not always recognize illness in themselves—or, if they do, they do not easily turn to others for help. Many feel guilty when things go wrong, and feel deeply ashamed when they do.

In this new edition of *The Medical Marriage*, Wayne and Mary Sotile gently shatter all the myths that surround the gamut of medical marriages. They address the universality of upheaval and stress in *all* marriages and give identity and hope to the countless medical couples who suffer in isolation. I guarantee that there is not a physician or a physician's spouse who will not be able to see him- or herself in one or more of the Sotiles' many vignettes, or who will not benefit from their many suggestions.

The Sotiles have been treating couples for over twenty years and are internationally respected experts and lecturers on physician marriages. Referring to the loneliness of many physician marriages, the authors state, "We are in the business of helping people meet the challenge of avoiding or escaping this miasma of 'quiet desperation.'" Indeed, they are. With this statement, they set the tone for the entire book. You will be engaged by their rich insights into your life as a physician, or as the spouse of a physician. They write with authority and a scholarly knowledge of the published literature on physician health, illness, and impairment. You will be struck by their understanding and compassion—and will benefit enormously from the profusion of tips that jumps from the pages. Their sensible advice is applicable to a range of physicians at all stages of marriage and in all branches of medicine.

A word about using this book: although easy to read, it is not for "lightweights." It is meaty and demanding. The Sotiles say "all hope is not lost" if your partner is not willing to participate in efforts to improve your relationship, but I suggest *strongly* that both of you tackle this book together. (I appeal here especially to men, whether you are a male physician or the husband of a physician; it is well known that men are a tough sell, and they do not tend to gravitate toward books on marriage!)

Here is what I say to medical couples at the end of my first visit with them: "You are making a very important statement to each other by coming to see me. That is, you care enough about each other and your relationship (and family) to give this priority in your busy lives. I'm glad that you're here together." Let me borrow from this: by reading this book together, you are demonstrating your commitment to your marriage and admitting that, like all humans, you have vulnerabilities and can learn from others.

I suggest that you work your way through the book, chapter by chapter, *together*; that you discuss the case examples with each other; that you answer the questions the authors pose; that you complete the questionnaires; and that you debate with each other the many points and suggestions. Let this book stimulate and renew your relationship.

The Sotiles ask in the conclusion of their book, Is making a medical marriage work really worth all this effort?" I think that you will answer "Yes!" Enjoy the journey.

Michael Myers, M.D.
Author, *Doctors' Marriages: A Look at the Problems and Their Solutions*

Acknowledgments

We thank the many people who make our own work/family juggling act so enjoyable:

• Kathy Hall, our administrative assistant and office manager—for living up to your former employer's recommendation: "The minute you hire Kathy Hall, your life will be at least 50 percent better than it was the minute before you hired her."

• Lynn Swaim, our typist—for your constant, loving reminders to not get lost in our ambitions.

• Joyce Waters, our secretary—for your caring attention to the details of our practice.

• Richard Martin, Elin Call, Lani Seltzer, Carol Walsh, Cleaver Hillman, Marie O'Hara, and Deidre Teasdale, our colleagues—for being the competent professionals and nice people you are. You have helped us to create the best, most pleasant practice in North Carolina.

• The many pharmaceutical companies and hospitals which continue to support educational programs that enhance the lives of physicians and their families—for putting your money where it truly makes a difference.

• The many medical societies, medical society alliances, specialty medical organizations, and hospital systems that have facilitated our work—for doing the right stuff to promote work/family balance for physicians in the new millenium.

• The great folks at the American Medical Association—for the compliment of partnering with us to create a book that makes us proud.

• Michael Meyers, M.D., for your pioneering and eloquent work to improve the quality of life of physicians. We admire you.

• Special thanks to J.D. Kinney, Acquisitions Editor for AMA Press—for believing in our work, for being willing to take a chance, and for your kind and astute guidance. We sincerely thank you, both for your insight and your friendship.

• And, most of all, to our daughters, Rebecca and Julia—for reminding us that the greatest heroes quietly make safe spaces for each other. Thanks for becoming young women we admire and cherish. We love each of you with our life.

Table of Contents

Introduction

The world breaks everyone. And afterward some are strong in the broken places.

—**Ernest Hemingway,** *A Farewell to Arms*

In order to become a physician, work as a physician, or live with a physician, you have to get used to an unusual level of stress. We know that no medical family needs a description of the stresses that come with a life in medicine; we assume that you might benefit, though, from help in understanding how to manage yourselves and your relationships as you face the challenges confronting medicine in modern times.

Neither of us is a physician. However, since 1979, we have collectively spent more than 60,000 hours observing countless high-powered marriages. We have counseled hundreds of physicians and their loved ones, both individually and as couples; thousands more have given us the privilege of working with them in workshop settings.

What we have learned is that thousands of medical couples are struggling to figure out how to juggle their work and family roles. The burning issue: How to create and maintain healthy relationships, at work and home.

Our work with physicians has taught us to appreciate an important fact: when a physician's personal relationships start to founder, the risks of professional disillusionment escalate. Furthermore, as professional disillusionment festers, marriage and home life are threatened. Conversely, stress resilience—defined as the ability to bounce back after being psychologically challenged—is promoted when physicians are able to establish and maintain reasonable, caring relationships with the people with whom they work and live.

Social researchers have documented that, for both men and women, an intimate marriage is a great boon to emotional and physical health and to work productivity. We have long known that supportive, intimate relationships can help you to better manage stress, improve your mood, and encourage healthy living. But we now also know that a loving, supportive marriage can increase work productivity and even decrease work absenteeism. Recent studies have shown that employees who have the benefit of helping behaviors and satisfaction in their marriages have fewer psychosomatic symptoms, less depression, and greater satisfaction with their jobs, even when the job is highly stressful.[1,2] Marital difficulties, on the other hand, seem to contribute to increased job turnover, general career dissatisfaction, and burnout.[3]

Building positive interpersonal cultures in the medical workplace is a focus of our consulting and research endeavors. Our thoughts on this topic are evolving as we work with individuals and groups in changing medical environments. Here, we want to focus on how physicians and their mates can shape positive marital dynamics. We will share both the lessons we have learned from medical families who have managed to avoid the major relationship potholes that fill the path of a medical couple, and our knowledge of what can be done to keep a long-term marriage functional *and* romantic. In the privacy of our counseling sessions, hundreds of variations on this theme have been raised:*

Sara, wife of a surgeon: *"Sometimes I feel like my husband doesn't even know me anymore. Here I am, pushing for more authenticity in all areas of my life, but he still seems to think that I'm the same naive 'young thing' he married during residency. That was seventeen years ago! What's worse is that now that I have grown up, he doesn't even seem interested in getting to know me."*

Ben, an internist: *"I've been committed to being an excellent physician since before I entered medical school. But I also want to be an excellent husband and father; I want a more reasonable balance between work and family than my medical mentors ever had. But I'm trapped: The senior physicians in my group think that I don't want to work enough, and my wife thinks I work too much."*

Betty, wife of an ophthalmologist: *"We went out to dinner last Friday, and I was crying before the soup was served. As I sat there in silence with my husband, noticing the animated conversations of other couples in the restaurant, I said, 'Let's talk.' His response shattered me: 'After this many years, what is there to talk about? We know each other's every thought, like, dislike, and hang-up. So what's new about an old relationship?'"*

Luke, a pathologist: *"I'm a 'rich doctor,' right? Then why do I lie awake nights trying to figure out how we can keep this lifestyle of ours afloat on less money? It costs more than we ever expected. Or maybe I'm just going to make less money than either of us ever dreamed I would."*

* All identifying information in case vignettes has been changed to protect the confidentiality of the individuals and couples described.

Audie, a pediatrician: *"I don't know why we never do the things that used to make us like each other: little surprises, saying 'please' and 'thank you,' saying nice things about each other in front of other people. I still feel like doing this stuff. But I just don't get around to it. I'm forever too tired or too angry or too preoccupied with one thing or another."*

Saul, an anesthesiologist: *"Overall, I'm satisfied with my life and my marriage. If I had it to do over again, I wouldn't change any major parts, even the ways that medicine has changed and is changing. But I secretly worry that we are just not growing as a couple. Maybe it's unrealistic to expect that you can stay interested and interesting in any single relationship over the long haul. But I sure do wish that we could find a way; my wife has been my best friend. The truth is, she's my only friend. I want her to remain my only lover."*

Karen, a psychiatrist: *"When we got together, we were both mature and experienced enough to understand that staying together would take work. We are both practicing psychiatrists; we spend our days helping other people get more realistic about their lives. But here we are, twelve years later, filled with resentments. We never dreamed that it would take this much work."*

A Few Sobering Facts

Fact: Approximately 50 percent of first-time marriages for those under the age of thirty-five end in divorce.[4]

Fact: As of 1999, nearly 40 percent of children under age eighteen did not live with their fathers.[5] Furthermore, recent research has shown that the belief that an unrewarding marriage should be ended may lead some people to invest less time in their marriages, make fewer attempts to resolve marital disappointments, and increase the odds of divorcing.[6]

Fact: Sweeping changes in medical economics, in how medicine is being practiced, and in the public image of physicians threaten the economic future and social position of physicians and their families. Perhaps this fact accounts for another statistic: More than 50 percent of practicing physicians say they would currently discourage future generations from entering their profession.[7]

Fact: Physicians under the age of forty-five consistently indicate that their most toxic stressor is struggle with work/family imbalance and its effect on home life.[8]

Fact: Research in England, Denmark, Scotland, and North America has documented that, compared to the general population, physicians and their spouses suffer significantly increased incidences of drug abuse, alcoholism, depression, thoughts of suicide, acts of suicide, and psychiatric hospitalizations.[9-13]

Fact: In addition to the classic stresses that have always bombarded medical couples (long work hours, little time for leisure, a high profile), contemporary medical couples seem to be struggling *with each other*. For example, the pioneers of medical marriage research, Glen Gabbard and Roy Menninger, claimed that physicians' long work hours don't *cause* their marital problems; instead, physicians' excessive work often *results from* their desire to escape marital tensions.[14]

Fact: Both clinical and empirical studies of physicians' marriages suggest that, despite their somewhat lower divorce rate, they tend to be less happy in their marriages than many others.[14]

Today's Medical Marriages

We seldom meet a medical couple who entered marriage prepared to face what was to come. Contemporary medical couples rank among the most stressed and surprised segment of the married population. A number of sweeping changes have helped shape these relationships. At work and home, medical families are facing more high-demand, low-control stress than ever before—the sort of stress that can prove toxic, rather than energizing.

The very structure of the "typical" medical marriage has also changed drastically. A household consisting of a physician devoted to the practice of medicine and a homemaker-wife who lovingly keeps the home running and the family happy—all the while gratified with her husband's accomplishments—is quickly becoming a thing of the past. These days, more than 60 percent of female spouses of physicians are employed outside the home.[15]

Those wives who are homemakers often view their physician-husbands in anything but a flattering light. Since the late 1970s, women's magazines have been publishing testimonials in which wives of physicians describe their mates as undemonstrative, cold, stilted, domineering, stern, compulsive, perfectionistic, and failures as husbands, fathers, and lovers. More recently, they have joined in the lament that the Marcus Welbys of yesteryear have now given way to a new breed of physicians who are driven, yet disillusioned with their profession and, often, with their lives.

Yet another change is shaking medical marriages: Between 1980 and 1997, the total number of women physicians increased 207.1 percent. Currently, more than 116,000 women are practicing medicine in the United States alone.[16] These women epitomize the dilemma faced by contemporary, female superachievers. Married or not, two thirds of female physicians juggle the roles of physician and mother. Many take full responsibility for running their homes and families while also working nearly as much in their profession as their male colleagues (most of whom have a nonphysician wife attending to their domestic life). When they do marry, women physicians tend to marry other physicians, and now, as always, when physicians marry each other, it is the woman who most often makes career sacrifices in deference to her family's needs.

If she does not marry another physician, a woman physician will almost always marry a professional. Regardless of how dynamic he is in his own right, the husband of a physician typically struggles with his version of the classic "physician's wife" syndrome: His career and marriage take a backseat to the status, prestige, income, and time demands of his wife's professional life. Many of these relationships are a cauldron of competition, anger, and tension over sex roles; these relationships often eventually produce an overfunctioning wife and an underfunctioning husband. What happens next is fascinating—and often tragic.

Many female physicians sabotage their own careers in an effort to recreate esteem for their foundering husbands, who are losing the "competition" within their marriage for status and prestige.

Even more sobering is a fact that suggests that the stresses of juggling career and family life seem to be especially detrimental to female physicians:

Fact: Until recently, women physicians were 40 percent more likely to divorce than their male colleagues.[17]

Stop Struggling and Get It Right

There is some good news: People today are fighting to save marriage. The great majority of Americans state that they want their marriage to last a lifetime.[18] And well they should.

Fact: Even after controlling for a variety of factors, the most well-conducted contemporary research indicates that an intact marriage in itself appears to make a positive difference in a child's well-being. Put another way, even when conflicting parents divorce, children are hurt *by the divorce itself.*[19]

In marriage, as in every human endeavor, there are always some people who manage to do what it takes to get the outcome they want, even when faced with circumstances that defeat others. A large percentage of the people we counsel manage to "get it right" when it comes to keeping romance in their marriage.

Fact: Over 60 percent of couples in intact marriages of thirty or more years report their marriages to be "very happy."[18]

In fact, for the most part, our clients have been exceptional people: successful, educated, and exceptionally capable of managing the stresses of their lifestyle. These people have impressed us with their abilities to use their resources to become successful in their work and their personal lives.

We want to describe these successful medical couples to you. The lessons that they have to teach can serve as beacons of hope and direction in the confusing times of change that face contemporary medical couples. Living testaments to the benefits of an intimate, passionate marriage, they seem to thrive, not struggle, as they move through the maze of a contemporary medical marriage with a style that is graceful, flexible, and obviously effective. They remind us of an important lesson: Stress is inevitable. Struggling is optional.

We first learned this lesson in Manhattan, where we were attending a workshop conducted by a respected psychotherapist. During the lunch break we walked six blocks to a deli, and as we were being seated, the therapist came in and joined us for lunch. As we walked back to the convention center, the three of us got caught in a summer rainstorm, and none of us had an umbrella. Two of us hunched over, resisting the buckets of water that were plastering our clothes and hair. After two blocks of this misery, our necks ached from scrunching, and our faces were cramped from grimacing at the unwanted dousing. Miserable and grouchy, we slogged along.

Finally, the conference center was in sight, and we sprinted the last thirty yards to the awning. After several minutes, we spotted the noted therapist leisurely strolling along, taking his time as he walked through the rain. Dripping and cursing our fate, we waited for him. Then we all entered the building. The therapist asked us a simple question: "When you get caught in a thunderstorm without an umbrella in North Carolina, does it help keep you *drier* if you scrunch up like that?"

Stress is inevitable.

Struggling is optional.

Will Your Marriage Survive Your Life?

The multiple roles, inflated expectations, and sheer amounts of stress faced by contemporary medical couples are abnormal. Whether you are a physician or the spouse of a physician, when it comes to the types and level of stress that fill your days, you must accept the fact that you are living an abnormal life. Living with this pressure fosters an elaborate system of beliefs, thoughts, and expectations that shape your personalities, both individually and as a couple. The coping patterns that emerge from such a stressful life can become a major complicating factor in keeping your marriage alive.

Beware of How You Cope

Stresses inherent in the lifestyles of most medical couples compel *both* mates—not just the physician—to develop self-focused styles of coping that carry one guarantee: Unless they are managed, misguided attempts to maintain control during the uncontrollable times that fill a medical marriage will damage the relationship to its core.

Fact: Partners in a medical marriage tend to cooperate in normalizing a lifestyle that sanctifies workaholism, competitiveness, controlling behavior, doing and thinking too many things at once, and generally living in a self-focused haze of hurry sickness. We call this the *super-couple syndrome*.[20]

Does This Apply to You?

Are you or your spouse stuck in styles of coping that risk damaging your marriage? To answer this question, take this *Have You Ever?* test. Honestly answer the following questions about yourself and about your partner:

Have you ever...

While stopped at a red light, spent the entire time looking at the green light for the opposite street, waiting tensely for that light to turn amber so that you can jam down your car's accelerator as soon as your light turns green?

Yes _____   No _____

Raced with the cars beside you to see who would win the privilege of being first at the next stoplight?

Yes _____   No _____

Questioned the heritage of another driver simply because the driver didn't know where he or she was going?

Yes _____   No _____

Found yourself rushing through some part of life (like eating lunch) for no good reason?

Yes _____   No _____

Reacted to a friendly game with a loved one or friend as though some important competition were at stake?

Yes _____   No _____

Fumed as you counted the items in the baskets of shoppers ahead of you in the express checkout line at the grocery store?

Yes _____   No _____

Managed to watch a single television show without checking what's on at least eight other channels?

Yes _____   No _____

Acted as though God appointed you "Official Finisher of Other People's Sentences" just to improve the "efficiency" of the conversation or "help out" lest someone forget what he or she is about to say?

Yes _____   No _____

Had difficulty not offering advice when someone was obviously only asking for support?

Yes _____   No _____

Spent more than three minutes doing absolutely nothing?

Yes _____   No _____

Had a charitable fantasy about why the elevator you were waiting for might be taking so long to arrive?

Yes _____   No _____

While waiting for an elevator to arrive, convinced yourself that the eight other people waiting for the elevator had probably been incompetent in their ability to press the elevator call button? (As in: "I think it would be best if I just gave this little button a push myself, given how incompetent the rest of the world is.")

Yes _____   No _____

Eaten your breakfast, read the morning paper, listened to CNN, looked over your upcoming day's schedule, and balanced your checkbook—all at once—while having "quality time" with your family?

Yes _____   No _____

While riding as a passenger, had trouble controlling your urge to blurt out, "Why don't you park here!" even when the driver was halfway into that very parking space?

Yes _____   No _____

In our experience, no couple can get through the above list without saying, at least once, "That describes me!" or "That describes you!" More than 10,000 professional articles about variations of these coping patterns have been published.[21] Amazingly, virtually no attention has been paid to the ways in which these psychological survival strategies—one or more of which we universally find in the couples we counsel—interplay with the dynamics of medical marriages.

Beware of Relationship Narcissism

The coping patterns that come with a high-powered life can lead to a form of relationship narcissism[22] that will complicate the course of medical marriage. This barrier to intimacy is not about self-aggrandizement; it's about stress. Let us elaborate.

It has been proposed that the majority of vital people living complex lives become "mature narcissists"—that is, preoccupied with their own anxieties, stresses, needs, and wants. Relationship narcissism does not refer to self-centeredness, vanity, self-admiration, or self-glorification, even though any of these factors may characterize a given individual's psychological makeup. Rather, the term *mature narcissist* refers to the relationship processes that accompany doing what needs to be done to cope in contemporary times. For physicians and their loved ones, this form of narcissism is not pathological. In fact, in many ways it is adaptive. As was explained by Christopher Lasch over a decade ago:

> Narcissism appears realistically to represent the best way of coping with the tensions and anxieties of modern life, and the prevailing social conditions therefore tend to bring out narcissistic traits that are present, in varying degrees, in everyone.[23]

Developing self-focused preoccupations is an almost inevitable result of one of three scenarios: becoming a physician, living as a physician, and living with a physician. In fact, a number of prominent researchers have suggested that the very factors that make people choose medicine as a career also predispose them to narcissism and propel them into lives filled with excessive work, trouble in intimate relationships, emotional struggle, poor self-care, and susceptibility to substance abuse and depression. Basically, this research theorizes that many individuals choose the medical profession out of misguided attempts to soothe narcissistic wounds.

British psychologist W. D. K. Johnson and the famous American physicians George Vaillant and Karl Menninger have all observed that a disproportionate number of physicians had childhoods lacking in nurturing attention.[12,24,25] As a result, many physicians spend a lifetime trying to soothe their emotional wounds by giving too much to others. Other physicians run from these same emotional wounds by assuming a stance of self-importance and omnipotence. In any case, such a person may become dependent on applause from others to maintain his or her wounded sense of self.

Even if you escaped such childhood pain, you did *not* avoid the rigors of medical training, medical practice, or living with someone who has gone through these. The words of physician Jack McCue apply to both physicians and their partners: "The education and training of physicians are gratuitously stressful and teach residents short-term adaptive behaviors that are, in the long run, maladaptive."[26]

While there is little doubt that working in medicine can lead to relationship narcissism, so, surprisingly, can being married to a physician. For both physician and spouse, being a caretaker of others offers an opportunity to give the care and attention that neither received as a child. For some physicians' spouses, grandiosity may be maintained through the idealization of, and identification with, the medical profession or with the role of physician's spouse.

The problem is that this process creates a fragile sense of self for *both* individuals. The relationship that evolves from such a dynamic is easily shattered. When the applause stops, or when the stresses involved in maintaining the stance of an all-giving caretaker lead to more disillusionment than gratification, the medical marriage founders. The resulting pain often increases obsessive self-focus and relationship narcissism.

Coping in the ways described in the *Have You Ever?* quiz above may help you survive the stress of your lifestyle. The problem is, living this way will ruin your most important relationships.

From listening to our clients, we are aware that medical couples are limited only by their ingenuity when it comes to concocting ways to combine stress reactions and relationship narcissism to erode marital intimacy.

Beth, wife of a urologist: *"It always has to be his way, or he refuses to be gracious—even if I coerce him into participating. Unfortunately, his way always has to do with his work: his schedule, his fatigue, his stress, his fears about the coming day."*

Bart, a urologist: *"I know that you have a headache. But my head aches worse than yours. I was up all night in the emergency room."* (So your headache doesn't count.)

Fred, a family-practice physician: *"I have always worked hard to get what I wanted, and I want you to look different than you do. So let's go on a diet together. If you discipline yourself, you can get back into your size 4 clothes."*

Maya, an otolaryngologist: *"I want to do the right thing, but I also want to be true to myself for a change. What's wrong with that? I've spent my life working hard and being responsible. I can't help it if I'm falling in love with someone else."*

Keith, husband of a surgeon: *"My extended family is more interesting than yours. I love your parents, but I just don't like being around them."*

Jason, husband of an obstetrician-gynecologist: *"Your past is a violation of our present. As far as I'm concerned, the less I know about how you were before we got together, the better off we will be."*

Megan, wife of a gastroenterologist: *"It's not enough for you to agree to do what I want to do. I'd like for you to want to do what I want to do."*

So What Can Be Done About All This?

Our clinical work with medical couples is straightforward and exceptionally effective. Here, as in the privacy of our offices, we begin with outright challenges to you that determine the necessary starting point of our work with any couple.

Challenge 1: Give up the myth of the balanced life.

As we will discuss shortly, many medical couples fall prey to the disillusionment that comes from buying into the belief that if they "wait until . . ." long enough, they will eventually attain the proverbial balanced life. Nothing could be further from the truth.

As we discussed in our book *Beat Stress Together: The BEST Way to a Passionate Marriage, a Healthy Family, and a Productive Life,*[20] this is the Beaver Cleaver family myth of the 1990s—an unrealistic yardstick that couples today use to evaluate themselves. It's a myth that carries only one guarantee: it will demoralize you.

Further, we propose that the term *balance* is often misconstrued to mean a static state of affairs, a final "perfect" solution in our role-juggling act. In truth, balance is a dynamic process, akin to the way we repeatedly adjust our course as we walk across a stream on slippery rocks. The real goals of balance are to support each other through periods of imbalance in work, marital, family, or individual concerns, and to take responsibility for remembering to regularly adjust course in order to attend to some heretofore neglected areas of life.

Challenge 2: You have the right to choose. So go ahead.

Decide whether or not you want to face what needs to be faced in order to keep your marriage alive or to resuscitate it if it's near death. You have a right to choose whether you want to stay together, enhance your relationship, and follow the program that we will outline.

We remind you that your marriage started with a commitment, and it will continue to grow into a mature romance only by recommitting— again and again—to the process of *making* it work. This notion of commitment seems to have fallen out of favor in recent years. Speaking of the political and psychological turmoil that have characterized recent decades, psychologist Marion Solomon warned:

> It is now clear that [this] turmoil . . . fostered an atmosphere that has been very damaging to relationships. Some important things were missing from the new psychologies. Commitment lost its virtue, as marriage came to be viewed as confining and detrimental to personal growth. Many believed that the ties that bind must be loosened and, if they interfered with personal development, cut.[22(p xii)]

Medical couples usually attain individual success by virtue of their ability to commit. They decide to maintain a certain standard of excellence in work, and they commit to doing what it takes to get the job done. They decide to maintain a certain level of physical fitness, and they commit to exercising regularly and eating healthily. They decide to attain a certain level of involvement in their communities, and they commit to volunteerism. If your marriage is to grow, you must learn to use this same tool at home. Once committed, you must learn to deal with another challenge.

Challenge 3: Acknowledge that when it comes to love and marriage, you will not be the exception to the rules.

Your talents and resources create many options for you. However, you *do not* have the option—no matter how capable you might be—to revitalize your marriage without working at it. It's a humbling fact, but it's a fact nonetheless: no matter how exceptional and unique you each are, if you are to grow as a couple, you each must learn to understand and accept some universals that apply to all intimate relationships. This means taking an honest look at your ways of coping with stress and dealing with each other.

Challenge 4: Begin now to use your best "stuff" to make your relationship better.

You gained your station and status in life by doing more than other people: You studied more, worked more, sacrificed more, and endured more. If you want to escape becoming one of those couples who are living together in semi-misery, *enduring* rather than *enjoying* their lives and each other, you'll have to do more for your marriage than they do for theirs. It takes work to escape what Marion Solomon labeled the infamous "withdrawn marriages" club. These couples remain united in the eyes of others but are haunted by the loneliness they feel within the privacy of their relationship:

> It seems that these spouses live together only for the sake of the children or for material advantage. Behind their restrained facade, both partners are watching and trying to control each other. . . . They have their work, their hobbies, their sports and their exercise. She feigns ignorance when he complains that she is not there emotionally, but he recognizes that he does the same to her. When they are not fighting, they live totally separate lives. He spends most of his time on the boat in the marina, where he has a whole separate group of friends. She is busy with her bridge and charity work (or her own career), which he avoids as much as possible. . . . They hate to be near one another. They make sure to have others join them when they go out to dinner or on vacation, because they have nothing to say to each other.[22(p34)]

We are in the business of helping people meet the challenge of avoiding or escaping this miasma of "quiet desperation."

In the pages that follow, we will present our thoughts and observations about relationships, just as we do in our private counseling sessions.

We will walk you through what we hope will be an enlightening and compassionate look at yourselves both as individuals and as a couple.

We will teach you how to pinpoint the individual and interactive steps of teamwork and overcome your awkwardness in learning new dances of intimacy.

We will describe how you can redirect your coping abilities so that your best skills fuel, rather than damage, your marriage and family life.

We will teach you the secrets of medical couples who thrive.

What if My Partner Won't Cooperate?

During any week of our professional lives, we encounter some version of a common scenario. One partner in a medical marriage schedules an appointment to discuss two things: (1) concern about their marriage and (2) pain that results from their spouse's unwillingness to attend counseling.

We know that not all successful people are open to receiving advice. After all, you *are* members of a group that tends to be exceptional: exceptionally independent, self-directed, private, and hardheaded. Given your life experience, it may seem reasonable to conclude that there is little of value to be learned from someone else about *your* most intimate relationships.

We also know that true growth in marriage requires cooperation. We hope that the information in this book will motivate both you and your spouse to work together in new ways that add zest, spice, and maturity to your relationship.

If you have a partner who is unwilling to participate in efforts to improve your relationship, all hope is not lost. Positive change in relationships most often starts with one person changing small things, such as your reactions during conflict, or your way of spending time and energy day to day. This either contributes to growth in a relationship or hastens its deterioration.

If you read this book in partnership, our hope is that our words will help stimulate your *individual* motivations to change. We want to help shape your choices. The most powerful choice available for creating and preserving the intimacy you desire is for *you* to redefine *your* role in the relationship. As Michele Weiner-Davis put it in her pragmatic book *Divorce Busting:*

> Relationships are such that if one person makes significant changes, the relationship must change. Too many marriages go down the drain because each spouse is waiting for the other to change first. . . . Change your marriage by changing yourself.[27]

The concepts that we offer in this book have proved to be effective in helping literally thousands of couples remain in love, regain their love, or at least understand what is happening to their partnership. We sincerely hope that our words will be helpful to you.

Good luck.

References

1. Azar B. Quelling today's conflict between home and work. *APA Monitor.* 1997;28:1, 16.

2. Lewis JM, Barnhart FD, Howard BL, Carson DI, Nace EP. Work stress in the lives of physicians. *Tex Med.* 1993;89:62-67. See also: Schwartzberg NS. Dual-earner families: the importance of work stress and family stress for psychological well-being. *J Occup Health Psychol.* 1999;1:211-233.

3. Greenglass ER, Fiksenbaum L, Burke RJ. The relationship betweeen social support and burnout over time in teachers. *J Soc Behav Pers.* 1994;9:219-230.

4. Council on Families. *Closed Hearts, Closed Minds: The Textbook Story of Marriage.* New York, NY: Institute for American Values; 1997.

5. US Bureau of the Census. *Marriage, Divorce, and Remarriage in the 1990s* (Current Population Reports, Tables M and N, 23-180). Washington, DC: US Bureau of the Census; 1991.

6. Amato PR, Rogers SJ. Do attitudes toward divorce affect marital quality? *J Fam Issues.* 1999;20:69-86.

7. Louis Harris Poll: Medical practice in the 1980s: physicians look at their changing profession, 1981. In: McCue J, ed. Doctors and stress: is there really a problem? *Hosp Pract.* 1986;21:11, 15-16.

8. Graham J, Ramirez AJ, Cull A, Finlay I, Hoy A, Richards MA. Job stress and satisfaction among palliative physicians. *Palliative Med.* 1996;10:185-194.

9. Heim E. Job stressors and coping in health professions. *Psychother Psychosom.* 1991;55:90-99.

10. Arnetz BB. White collar stress: what studies of physicians can teach us. *Psychother Psychosom.* 1991;55:197-200.

11. Domenighetti G, Tomamichael M, Gutzwiller F, Berthoud S, Casabianca A. Psychoactive drug use among medical doctors is higher than in the general population. *Soc Sci Med.* 1991;33:269-274.

12. Johnson WDK. Predisposition to emotional distress and psychiatric illness amongst doctors: the role of unconscious and experimental factors. *Br J Med Psychol.* 1991;64:317-329.

13. Lawrence JM. Stress problems in the medical profession. *Aust Fam Phys.* 1989;18:1379-1389.

14. Gabbard GO, Menninger RW. The psychology of postponement in the medical marriage. *JAMA.* 1989;262:2378-2381.

15. Moore EE. Presidential address: swimming with the sharks without the family being eaten alive. *Surgery.* 1990;108:125-138.

16. Pasko T, Seidman B. *Physician Characteristics and Distribution in the US.* Chicago, Ill: American Medical Association;1999:12-13.

17. Roscow I, Rose KD. Divorce among doctors. *J Marriage Fam.* 1972;34:587-598.

18. Council on Families in America. *Marriage in America: A Report to the Nation.* New York, NY: Institute for American Values; 1995.

19. Spruijt E, de Goede M. Transitions in family structure and adolescent well-being. *Adolescence.* 1997;32:897-911.

20. Sotile WM, Sotile MO. *Beat Stress Together: The BEST Way to a Passionate Marriage, a Healthy Family, and a Productive Life*. New York, NY: John Wiley & Sons; 1999.
21. Williams R. *The Trusting Heart: Great News About Type A Behavior*. New York, NY: Time Books; 1989.
22. Solomon M. *Narcissism and Intimacy: Love and Marriage in an Age of Confusion*. New York, NY: WW Norton; 1989.
23. Lasch C. *The Culture of Narcissism: American Life in An Age of Diminishing Expectations*. New York, NY: Warner Books; 1979:101.
24. Menninger K. Psychological factors in the choice of medicine as a profession. *Bull Menninger Clin*. 1957;21:51-58, 99-106.
25. Vaillant GE, Sobowale NC, McArthur C. Some psychological vulnerabilities of physicians. *N Engl J Med*. 1992;287:372-375.
26. McCue J. Doctors and stress: is there really a problem? *Hosp Pract*. 1986;21:11, 15-16:15.
27. Weiner-Davis M. *Divorce Busting*. New York, NY: Fireside, 1992.

Further Reading

For information regarding the health benefits of a marriage, see:

Gove W, Style CB, Hughes M. The effect of marriage on the well-being of adults. *J Fam Issues*. 1990;27:233-250.

Hu Y, Goldman N. Mortality differences by marital status: an international comparison. *Demography*. 1990;27:233-250.

Kiecolt-Glaser JK, Fisher LD, Ogrocki P, Stout JC, Speivher CE, Glaser R. Marital quality, marital disruption, and immune function. *Psychosom Med*. 1987;49:13-34.

Lillard LA, Waite LJ. Til death do us part: marital disruption and mortality. *Am J Sociol*. 1995;100:1131-1156.

Waite LJ. Does marriage matter? *Demography*. 1995;32:483-507.

Wilson BF, Schoenborn C. A healthy marriage: does marriage foster a healthy lifestyle, or do healthy people get married? *Am Demographics*. 1989:40-43.

For information regarding work productivity and marital/family relationships, see:

Azar B. Quelling today's conflict between home and work. *APA Monitor*. 1997;28:1, 16.

Burke RJ, Weir T. Marital helping relationships: the moderators between stress and well-being. *J Psychol*. 1977;95:121-130.

Coyne JC, DeLongis A. Going beyond social support: the role of social relationships in adaptation. *J Consult Clin Psychol*. 1986;54:454-460.

Greenglass ER, Fiksenbaum L, Burke RJ. The relationship between social support and burnout over time in teachers. *J Soc Behav Personality*. 1994;9:219-230.

Hendrix WH, Spencer BA, Gibson GS. Organizational and extraorganizational factors affecting stress, employee well-being, and absenteeism for males and females. *J Business Psychol*. 1994;9:103-128.

Schultz JB, Henderson C. Family satisfaction and job performance: implications for career development. Special Issue: Family-career linkages. *J Career Dev.* 1985;12:33-47.

Weisman CS, Teitelbaum MA. The work-family role system and physician productivity. *J Health Soc Behav.* 1987;28:247-257.

Yandoli AH. Stress and medical marriages. *Stress Med.* 1989;5:213-219.

For discussion of high-demand, low-control stress, see:
Karasek R. *Healthy Work.* New York, NY: Basic Books; 1992.

Regarding the effect of divorce on children, see:
Booth A, Dunn J, eds. *Stepfamilies: Who Benefits? Who Does Not?* Hillsdale, NJ: Lawrence Erlbaum; 1994.

McLanahan S, Sandefur G. *Growing Up With a Single Parent.* Cambridge, Mass: Harvard University Press; 1994.

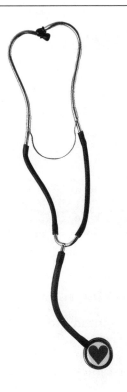

Part 1

Stress, Personality, and Marriage

Chapter 1

Beating Stress Together

*We need not so much to be taught as to
be reminded.*

—C. S. Lewis

That medical marriages are stressful is not news. We all know that we are living in a stress epidemic that threatens our physical, emotional, and family health. What we don't always notice is the effects of this stress on our personal lives.

The Prize for Being (or Marrying) a Physician

Nearly three decades of research have indicated that, compared to such fellow professionals as attorneys and dentists, physicians are at higher risk for emotional, physical, and relationship ailments. These elevated risks exist throughout the physician's career, from the earliest days of medical school until retirement.

Fact: Approximately 40 percent of female and 27 percent of male medical students and residents experience pronounced symptoms of anxiety or depression.[1]

Fact: Compared to controls, medical residents are five and one-half times more likely to use sleeping pills, stimulants, and other drugs.[2] These statistics are understandable, given the intense, exhausting, and critical nature of medical education and training. But it is also true that symptoms of distress do not stop upon completion of medical training. In fact, they usually get worse. The high stress of medical life, coupled with the availability of drugs, leads a disproportionate number of physicians into the "rollerball" syndrome: The stresses of their life jack them up throughout the day, leading to the use of tranquilizers during the day and sleeping pills at night.

Fact: Worldwide research has indicated that the rate of drug dependence for physicians is somewhere between thirty and 100 times greater than for the general population.[3,4] Research of physician rates of alcohol abuse is somewhat controversial. Some studies have indicated that physicians suffer from alcoholism two and one-half times more frequently than other members of their socioeconomic class.[5] More recent research suggests rates of alcohol abuse for physicians ranging between 13 and 14 percent.[6] This rate is consistent with the 13.5 percent rate of alcohol disorders in the adult population.[7] However, physicians do suffer more from certain illnesses and die younger from certain causes.

Fact: Compared to the general population, physicians suffer greater incidences of cardiovascular disorders, leukemia, and cirrhosis.[8] Research from Finland, Britain, Japan, Denmark, and the United States has also shown that the all-cause mortality rates of physicians are higher than those for all other professionals combined.[9]

The prevalence of such illnesses, coupled with the fact that physicians have a significantly higher rate of suicide than age-matched cohorts, leads to yet another noteworthy observation.

Fact: While physicians have a slightly longer life span than the average person, they actually die younger than those from socioeconomically comparable groups.[8] In fact, some researchers have found that, while the average woman lives approximately ten years longer than the average man, the average female physician lives *ten years fewer* than the average male physician.[9]

The good news? Research is demonstrating that it is *not* necessarily true that stress is harmful. To the contrary, many people actually thrive while living high-stress lives. These are the people who manage to beat stress together.

Beat Stress Together

Our *Beat Stress Together (BEST)*[10] model centers on avoiding a classic mistake made by many dynamic individuals who misuse their considerable talents when it comes to dealing with stresses and emotions. These people acclimate to toxic environments and ways of managing stress rather than changing things to live life in a more self-nurturing way. In short, they confuse the concepts of *noble* and *normal*.

We believe that a wealth of coping strength actually predisposes you to making a fundamental stress-management mistake: Because of your exceptional coping abilities, you are at risk of normalizing what is essentially an abnormal way of living. No matter how stressed you get, you are capable of going numb and pressing on.

These days, life is filled with abnormal kinds and levels of stress. Remember, the "normal" human stress scenario used to go something like this:

"Okay. The sun's up. We need to go kill a rabbit or pick some corn before the sun goes down. Come on, family! Let's go outside and do this together!"

To accomplish their daily tasks, families, as teams, spent time together outdoors: working, smelling the fresh air, noticing the changing seasons, probably even pausing occasionally to play in the clover or take a dip in a pond or mountain stream.

Of course, this is a rather simplistic and romanticized picture of what life was like during earlier times. But even during difficult periods, the typical lifestyle of earlier generations contained inherent stress management activities—physical exercise, interacting with nature, and family and community support.

Consider a typical stress scenario in a medical marriage:

Partner 1: *Oh, boy! I'm exhausted. I woke up with a headache. I was at the ER until 2:30 this morning, and then I couldn't sleep. But I have a full day—committee meetings and office hours this morning and surgery this afternoon. No time to wimp out. I can't afford to be tired today.*

I need to hurry. I've got to stop by the hospital and cast my vote about hiring or firing several colleagues, then get to my office. I'll be late, as usual. But I'd better run by the bank on my way, because we are in 'ready reserve' for the third time this month.

Partner 2: *(an annoyed look)*

Partner 1: *You have that look in your eyes. I hate that look. What did I do? Yesterday wasn't my day to pick the kids up from after-school sports. You do that on Tuesdays, Thursdays, and Fridays. So what did I miss? The ball game? I forgot our son's ball game! Darn! Why didn't you remind me? I can't help it if I had a day filled with chaos. Don't look at me like that. It's not exactly like I'm having fun here.* (Phone rings.)

Partner 2: *It's your answering service. I've got to go; I have my own meetings—and my own headache—today.*

When you consider all the stress faced by contemporary medical couples, you might deem such a lifestyle *noble*, but living this way is not *normal*.

Keys to *BEST*

Effective emotional managers use their skills to do what they can do to create a nurturing and affirming life territory. By "territory," we mean the arenas in which you live your life. These are created by the *situations*, *processes*, and *relationships* that fill your life. To do your BEST, you must ensure that your boundaries have no holes; your situations, processes, and relationships must be fundamentally nurturing and affirming. Within this territory, effective emotional managers fill their lives, as much as possible, with what stress researchers Suzanne Kobasa and colleagues call the "three *C*s" of stress-hardiness: involvements that *challenge* them, to which they are *committed*, and over which they have some sense of *control*.[11] In this regard, stress-hardy people manage their lives by managing themselves. They manage stress from the inside out, using their attitudes, coping tendencies, and relationship dynamics as a way of maintaining control of their overall emotional well-being.

Your life arenas are defined by three factors:

1. Your life *situations* include the places in which you spend time: work setting, community, clubs, place of worship—wherever you live your life. In other words, situations are your life's *where* factor.

2. By *processes*, we mean the ways in which you treat yourself. This is your *how* factor: how you label yourself, how you treat your body, how you manage your spiritual life and your coping patterns. Processes are the general choices you make in orchestrating your life.

3. By *relationships*, we mean, of course, the people in your life, or your *who* factor: whom you fill your life with, and how you manage those relationships. This life arena includes your spouse, family, friends, and acquaintances. Here, as in all aspects of our *BEST* model, we focus on ways you can better control the outcomes that affect you. Rather than focusing on what other people do *to* you, learn to use your own skills to generate the relationship outcomes that you want.

It's Not as Simple as It Sounds

If you are to thrive, you must regularly evaluate the situations, processes, and relationships that structure your life and examine your life from the perspective of the three *C*s of stress hardiness. For most medical couples, doing so may at first lead to painful feelings—specifically, loss, outrage, and longing.

For many medical couples, the process of evaluation usually means dealing with feelings of loss for what was—or is being—missed because of grueling work schedules that interfere with loving and nurturing contact with each other. Two brief case examples demonstrate this process.

We once treated a young neurosurgeon who was coerced into seeking our help when his wife threatened to divorce him after he slapped her in the middle of one of their frequent arguments. Faced with the trauma that his wife might leave him and that she was seriously questioning whether she still loved him, the man crumbled. What poured forth was a flood of emotions that had boiled inside him, fueling both his ambition and his rage:

Yeah, I guess you're right: I do tend to go numb and store up anger. Let me explain it to you; let me make it perfectly clear: I'm thirty-five years old, and I've been in school or training for thirty-one of those years, counting kindergarten. Somewhere along the way of residency, I learned to go 'numb.' What else was I supposed to do? Have you ever been on call every other night for years in a row? Do you know what it feels like never to see your family, to spend every holiday with a pit of anxiety in your stomach or feeling exhausted? Do you know what it feels like to be saving other people's lives but losing your own life—your own family?

You're darned right I'm angry! My wife is wounded by the facts of our life, facts that she remembers like an elephant. I wasn't there when our son was born. I missed his first birthday party. Umpteen times I have had to eat holiday meals on the run. I forgot our wedding anniversary once. We don't have sex as often as we used to. I sometimes fall asleep while we're supposedly 'out on a date.' If I'm awake, I'm preoccupied. And on and on and on!

Well, I've got a memory, too. That was my little boy being born while I was out moonlighting. (Crying now) *That was my son having his first birthday while I was stuck in the OR for seventeen hours, inside some suicide victim's head, all the while being harassed by that sadistic attending who acted like I was the one who blew half of this patient's brains out. I'm the one who can't remember feeling like I deserved to take time off to enjoy my holidays or my family or my life!*

(Regaining composure) *I come home these days and don't even know what my wife is angry about. That's what drives me most crazy. I don't have a clue. I just know she's angry with me. I guess she's still angry about my forgetting our anniversary. I didn't mean to. I was in the middle of studying for my boards, and I just forgot. I can't find any relief anywhere I go.*

As you honestly evaluate your feelings and attitudes, you may also notice outrage at the very institution of medicine for its intrusion into the privacy of your life. Beyond the outrage, you are also likely to long for what you still do not get enough of. The comments of Ellen, the wife of a urologist, typified both of these points.

I'm here because of my headaches, which my doctor tells me are due to hypertension. I don't need you to tell me what's driving up my blood pressure. Let me tell you: the pressure is coming from the anger in my heart. I am the loneliest forty-one-year-old woman I know. My husband was basically absent during the first three years of our marriage because he was completing his residency. I kept my sanity during those years by staying angry at the director of his residency. I blamed that man for the pain in my heart; he was the one who intimidated my husband into being gone all the time.

Now he's in practice, scrambling to make money while the sun is still shining somewhat on medicine, and the scramble is keeping him gone from home all the time. I blame the other partners in his group for scaring him into believing that this is necessary. I blame the director of the HMO that is taking over our town and his practice, and I blame the politicians for keeping my husband the wreck that he became as he learned how to be a physician.

I used to blame my husband, but now I just see him as a victim of all of this. I just want him to be with me more often; not just physically but also with his interest and his energy. I want his presence—that vibrant, enthusiastic presence that swept me off my feet so many years ago.

Sometimes when I look at him I feel like crying. He's getting that glazed-over, numb look that we used to joke about seeing on the faces of all of those 'old men' faculty at his medical school. I'm scared of what is happening to him and to us, and I don't believe that this is going to stop.

Stress Resilience

The most fundamental way of examining the stress in your life is to ask a simple question: "When it comes to meeting *my* needs, is the territory of my life mostly toxic or mostly nurturing?" By *toxic*, we mean anything that makes you feel anxious, frightened, miserable, or generally uncomfortable. By *nurturing*, we mean anything that makes you feel reasonably secure, appreciated, and acknowledged.

> **Fact:** Rather than being a positive and reinforcing experience, medical training often functions as a "colossal castrator for the unwary student."[12]

Recently, the findings of several major studies[13,14] set off alarms throughout the world of academic medicine and induced knowing nods during private conversations between physicians and their loved ones. These studies called attention to how frequently medical students and residents suffer psychological and physical abuse at the hands of their superiors. As many as 80 percent of medical students surveyed reported having been verbally attacked, and 24 percent claimed that they suffered physical abuse (being slapped, kicked, or hit, or having things thrown at them) during their training. These figures did *not* include the norm of subjecting medical residents to inhumane periods of sleep deprivation. The students who were surveyed claimed that it is commonplace to function on as little as twenty-eight hours of sleep per week and that periods of work-filled sleeplessness may range from thirty to 100 hours. Furthermore, 81 percent of women physicians in training reported being sexually harassed or mistreated by clinical faculty, senior residents, or superior interns, and 50 percent of Latino students and residents reported suffering racial harassment or discrimination.

The stress onslaught does not end upon completion of medical education. Once in the "real world," medical couples encounter various flavors of stress—some clear, others subtle.

Fact: On average, male physicians work between sixty-eight and eighty hours per week. Married female physicians, in addition to taking major responsibility for home and family, work 90 percent as much as their male colleagues.[15,16]

When your life is filled with either toxic stress or overwhelming amounts of stress, the outcome is clear: you *will* be distressed, and the goal is to endure. This situation is painful but not confusing. More frightening is the situation in which dissatisfaction fills your days for reasons that are not apparent to you. Jake Landry was a case in point.

Jake Landry was a person who always excelled. Things came easily to him. He soared through high school, basking in the glory of being a star athlete and an outstanding student. In college, chemistry and physics were as much his hobbies as his major courses of study. Medical school was challenging but not intimidating to Jake, and his residency and fellowship in infectious diseases represented a highlight in his quest to become a physician and a medical scientist.

It was also during residency that Jake met Patrice. They married as Jake completed his medical training, and the two of them settled into a comfortable but fast-paced life that revolved around Jake's immersion in his first job in academic medicine and Patrice's work as a junior–high-school teacher. During the initial stages of his career and his marriage, all went well and as planned. Jake thrived in academia and especially loved the intellectual challenges and stimulation of medical research and teaching.

The Landrys even had their children as planned: one son and one daughter, spaced three years apart. Patrice willingly suspended her teaching career in order to focus on home and hearth, and for the first seventeen years of their marriage, the Landrys created an exceptionally stable and comfortable lifestyle.

As their children entered early adolescence, Jake and Patrice grew concerned about finances. Faced with the changes in national health care in the mid-1980s, they reasoned that they should focus on maximizing their income during the next decade in order to safeguard their financial future. Patrice considered returning to teaching, but instead she and Jake decided that he should leave his medical school faculty position and enter the more lucrative world of private practice. Jake created a burgeoning practice, nearly doubling his income within four years.

The Landrys enjoyed the fruits of this sudden boon in income. They bought a new house, funded their kids' educational trust, created a lucrative retirement plan, and joined a country club. The Landrys seemed to be thriving—except for one problem. Jake began acting progressively more depressed and irritable. He frequently withdrew from Patrice and their children, especially when Patrice expressed concern that Jake was drinking to excess.

Jake never would have consulted us had his wife not coerced him into doing so. But it was also true that Jake entered our offices with worries of his own. In fact, he shared Patrice's concerns, but was confused about what to do about them. He stated,

"I've created a monster in this practice. I work more and more, but what am I supposed to do? The practice is only five years old, and I'm making good money. Plus I have sick patients and limited help. Being in practice means working hard, and Patrice needs to learn how to tolerate it. We both knew this would be the deal when we decided that I'd make this move."

Even though he wouldn't admit it to his wife, Jake was also concerned about his drinking:

"I don't know what the deal is between me and alcohol. Patrice and I have always been social drinkers. Everyone I know drinks. What bothers me is that the only time I come close to relaxing is after three scotches. I know enough medical facts about alcohol to fear what I see. I don't feel pleasure unless I'm half-looped. My endorphins just aren't flowing the way they used to when I jogged regularly. Problem is, I don't have time to jog. I'm exhausted half the time and angry the other half. If I want to have fun, I need some help to make it happen in a hurry."

Yet another concern of Jake's was that he found himself constantly fantasizing.

"I fantasize about everything. At least that's how it seems. I think about other women. I think about another life. I think about how it used to be for me professionally. I think about how it must be for other people. I use three-fourths of my brain to think about everything under the sun and the other fourth to get through my life."

Jake was especially bothered and confused by his fantasizing because he saw this as a sign of dissatisfaction with his life. In his words:

"I'm careful not to insult myself by acting like a middle-aged man taking his turn at trying to screw up his life. I swear, I don't know why I'm doing this. I love Patrice. Our sex life has always been as good as I would let it be, given my fatigue and moodiness. I don't know, I just feel irritated, and she seems to be the one irritating me by being so 'normal' and happy with our life. Half the time I feel like screaming. But I can't even say why."

As we got to know this honest man, the complexity of his inner struggles began to make sense. We asked him to talk more about his fantasies.

"The truth is, I'm constantly living as an observer—I watch myself go through the motions. What I'm observing is how little of myself is 'into' what I do day to day.

"*Last Thursday night, as usual, we went to family grill night at our club. I felt depersonalized the whole evening, like a part of me was observing me and my family go through the motions of seeing the same old people we see every Thursday night and having the same old banter we have with the same old couples. What scared me was how phony I felt and how satisfied my wife looked. I know what you're going to say— she's not the problem here. I know that. The problem is, I don't know what the problem is. I just know that I'm not very happy and that I'm getting symptomatic.*

"*Don't get me wrong; I'm not casting stones. I like my neighborhood, and I appreciate the good things that fill our life. My kids are secure, our home is beautiful, the people we associate with are decent and good. I'm just bored. We go through the same routines with the same people month after month. My problem is that I'm not willing to upset the apple cart. Patrice enjoys this. Her only problem is my dissatisfaction.*

"*I have similar feelings about my career. I see patients and treat their illnesses, but I don't get that charge or that sweet obsession about ideas and medical concepts and medical questions and possible answers like I used to when I was in academia. When I left the medical school, I vowed that I would keep some form of research going, but I haven't. Now I plow through my days, seeing patient after patient, doing nothing to enhance my mind or medical knowledge. I feel like a user of, rather than a contributor to, medical science. Some guys are satisfied being practitioners; I'm not.*

"*I'm also tired of my friends. Everything I do is pressured. I see the same guys and do the same things with them month after month. We play poker and golf, and we talk sports. I enjoy these things, but they all have a common theme—competition. I'm tired of competition. I was thinking about this the other day, and I got depressed. All my life I've been competing. For example, I love my three brothers, but all we ever did was compete—at sports, in academics, in our careers, everywhere. I built a life around excelling. I had to excel in order to get into college, get into medical school, get out of medical school, get into residency, get out of residency, get my first job, get promoted, and then to get into practice. Now I'm constantly competing to solidify my practice. Does it ever stop? I don't think I've ever had a relationship with another man that was not based on some form of friendly or not-so-friendly competition.*

"*Sometimes I just want to break away. I want to get more involved in research and less in clinical practice. I'd like for Patrice and myself to meet people who know and do different things. I want us to do different things, to break out of our mold. We see ads for vacations we'd like to take or plays we'd like to see, but we never go. We run across interesting people who are outside of our immediate neighborhood and social circle, but we never get to know them.*

"Sometimes I try talking with Patrice about this, but either it doesn't come out right or she just doesn't want to hear it. Her response is: 'What in the world are you talking about? We need to wait until the kids are educated and on their own, and then we'll be able to do whatever we want. Until then, look on the bright side.'

"I feel like I've created this big life and that I'm disappearing in it."

We repeat: The most fundamental way to examine the stress of your life is to ask a simple question. Is the territory of my life more toxic or nurturing to me?

Think about the situations, processes, and relationships that define Jake Landry's life. His life *situations* are reasonable: good job, good club, good community. In general, however, his life situations do not challenge him or satisfy his need for variety.

His *relationships* are sound, but not intimate. He loves his wife and kids. He basically likes his friends, but he is tired of the constant theme of competition. He is not growing in these relationships. Instead, he is observing himself playing various roles and is not open and involved with the people around him. He doesn't act on his natural curiosity and interest in new people.

Most obviously, the *processes* of Jake's lifestyle are causing him pain. He spends his energy observing himself becoming stagnant. He is plagued with self-questioning and self-criticism. His actions are not aligned with his inner thoughts, feelings, needs, or wants. He fantasizes about a different life but does nothing to initiate change. Most painful is Jake's growing habit of discounting his own accomplishments. He constantly notices all that he is *not* and all that he has *not* done and only halfheartedly notes the positive choices in his life.

Our practice is filled with people who share their version of Jake Landry's story. They see nothing major wrong with their lives, but feel unfulfilled. They lament their loss of motivation to continue with what used to give their lives meaning: getting educated, finding a partner to love, establishing a nice life, getting promoted, or creating a family. They lose their passion.

Much of Jake Landry's discontent came, not from stress, but from struggling to remain stuck in the same lifestyle, even though he regularly felt pangs of motivation to do something different.

Often the longings for a different way of life begin as relatively small stirrings—curiosity about a new movie or acquaintance or work routine. But the Landrys fell into "postponement," a phenomenon that was first explored by Glen Gabbard and Roy Menninger in their scholarly book *Medical Marriages.*[17] Postponement occurs when a medical couple grow accustomed to living a life of waiting. They pin their hopes of eventually getting around to enjoying their life and relationship upon the completion of the current quest:

"Once I complete this stage of my training, then I'll start spending some quality time with my loved ones."

"Once we get accustomed to this new practice, then we'll be able to enjoy our life together."

"Once we repay all of these debts, then we'll start feeling successful."

"Once the kids grow up and stop annoying me, then I'll enjoy parenting them."

Postponement can become a very dangerous habit. As the years progress, couples who live this way often place attending to their relationship lower and lower on their list of priorities. They become disconnected from each other and lose their intimacy—and often their friendship.

Gabbard and Menninger claim that this postponement lifestyle is a double-edged sword. On the one hand, it gives meaning to life when physicians must delay gratification while going through medical education and training. On the other hand, it allows people who are not comfortable in their relationship to continue avoiding the anxiety that comes from trying to maintain closeness with loved ones. Such individuals avoid their area of relative incompetence by constantly filling life with reasons to continue "waiting until."

The bustle of most medical couples' lives makes postponement a hard trap to avoid. As life goes on, a physician actually tends to be less involved in family life, not more.

Fact: A study of parenting stress involving spouses of male residents and house staff found that 75 percent of staff spouses expected parenting stress to decrease after residency, but 50 percent reported that stress actually *increased* when their mates ended residency. Only 25 percent stated that the level of stress had remained about the same.[18]

As we will discuss in chapter seven, some couples postpone cleaning up their life territory and rejoining each other until the later years of their marriage. For some, the second half of marriage comes as a welcome relief. Others find that they've waited too long; they lost each other on the journey.

Where to Begin: Ending the "Conspiracy of Silence"

Searching for external causes of stress will only make you miserable and will not improve your marriage. Instead, you must take an honest look at the inner workings of your psyches and partnership.

The causes of stress in the lives of vigorous people, physicians included, are often misunderstood. More important in determining stress hardiness or stress victimization are the interpersonal consequences of your respective personality-based cognitive and behavioral coping tendencies.

Many competent people, especially health professionals, complicate their lives by failing to identify the role these play in generating interpersonal circumstances that complicate their own stress symptoms.

Fact: Most high-powered people deny that all of the above applies to them.

Such denial leads to what Jack McCue calls the "conspiracy of silence"[19(pp7-16)] that physicians and their loved ones perpetuate: "Within our profession there is a reluctance to discuss the stresses of medical practice and, worse yet, an unwillingness even to acknowledge their existence."[19(p7)] The consequences sometimes spiral physicians into dangerous suffering contests.

During a recent consultation to a major medical training institution, we encouraged senior faculty and residents to openly discuss their work/family issues. Residents repeatedly voiced the belief that their personal relationships would improve upon completion of training. Senior faculty repeatedly cautioned that relationship tensions don't end automatically with graduation; competition among colleagues may continue to drive work/family imbalance.

The senior faculty were soon embroiled in a frank discussion about the subtle ways they attribute status to each other based on self-sacrificing, workaholic behavior. The faculty parking deck was identified as being one arena for earning such kudos. Faculty whose vehicles appeared earliest and remained latest each day in the parking deck were subtly acknowledged as being heroically dedicated to their profession.

As they discussed the absurdity of this competition, one faculty member sheepishly admitted, "I sometimes leave my third car in the lot for a week at a time, just to impress the rest of you."

Pressures like this can leave medical couples isolated and lead to symptom-producing attempts at solving the problems that come with a medical life. Caught between unrealistic and unrelenting time demands from work and home, and facing implied or stated criticism that they are falling short in one or both arenas, many physicians drift into an embarrassed state of withdrawal that is masked with anger or seeming indifference to their relationships in both arenas.

Alan, a forty-three-year-old radiologist, was referred for anger management counseling after a series of temper outbursts directed at nursing staff resulted in his being disciplined by hospital administration. He was clearly caught in a web of tensions at work and at home that drained his patience and coping reserves.

"This all started when I took a 30 percent cut in pay after our hospital forced the purchase of our practice. As if that weren't bad enough, I then had to increase my work hours to satisfy my new contract. Neither

of those things went over very well at home. My wife and I have been struggling about her plan to return to her work as a nurse. After ten years of staying home to raise our kids, I guess she deserves to get back into her profession. I can't argue against that. But she's being unrealistic about it: She says that it's my turn to take over some of the home responsibilities and facilitate her *career, just like she did for me.*

"My response? Go tell it to the hospital administrator, the same one who now owns my career. If I don't work, I lose my job."

Alan admitted that, as his marital conflict escalated, he found it *increasingly difficult to tolerate "incompetence in that hospital." He also admitted that he was daunted by the complex relationships that filled his life.*

"Look, I'm a person who's never really been comfortable dealing with conflict. Now, my life is filled *with conflict-filled relationships. This is like a nightmare! I'll tell you, I have a lot of fantasies about just walking—out of this marriage, this town, and this profession. This just isn't what I bargained for."*

What happens next to medical couples affected by these all-too-familiar stressors can be tragic. Emotional withdrawal leads to a retreat from family life and an unwillingness and inability to share feelings and experiences. Social isolation increases as the years pass, and as the pain mounts, so does the denial of its existence. The result is a relationship filled with moodiness, fatigue, work, loneliness, and, eventually, two distressed mates.

Fact: Women in dual-earner couples report increased depression when their mates withdraw from actively sharing responsibility for running their homes.[20,21]

Fact: Cutting-edge research with dual-earner couples has found that family stress is more important in determining depression for fathers than mothers.[20]

Ending this conspiracy of silence starts in the privacy of your dialogue with your mate and continues in your dealings with colleagues. This dialogue should *not* be a litany of how your mate has been frustrating you, but an honest disclosure of your own inner workings and the effect these are having on the situations and relationships that structure your life. The keys to beating stress together are to take control of that which is controllable and to be reasonable. It takes courage to stop surrounding yourself with toxic situations, relationships, and processes. Behaving in ways that will fulfill your inner needs and filling your life with situations, relationships, and processes that *reasonably* satisfy your needs for commitment, challenge, and control are what *BEST* is all about.

No one is able to create and maintain a perfectly nurturing life. For most of us, managing a stress-hardy life is difficult work. We must constantly adjust our reactions—and the people and places that comprise our territory—to ensure that we do not settle for what is essentially a toxic, unhealthy lifestyle.

You are fortunate if, naturally and spontaneously, your day-to-day life is filled with involvements that you are challenged by, committed to, and in control of. For most, these three Cs are *created*; they don't appear spontaneously. You may have to alter your perspective so that a given day's activity (or stage of life) has three *C* meaning. Alternatively, you may have to change activities so that your days are filled with a fair share of meaningful challenges. You may also have to learn new skills in order to increase your sense of control as you face these challenges.

None of this is possible without taking an honest look at what is causing your stress.

References

1. Hendrie HC, Clair DK, Brittain HM, Fadul PE. A study of anxiety/depressive symptoms of medical students, house staff, and their spouses/partners. *J Nerv Ment Dis.* 1990;178:204-207.
2. Myers T, Weiss E. Substance use by interns and residents: an analysis of personal, social, and professional differences. *Br J Addict.* 1987;82:1091-1099.
3. Rucinski J, Cybulska E. Mentally ill doctors. *Br J Hosp Med.* 1985;33:90-94.
4. Domenighetti G, Tomamichael M, Gutzwiller F, Berthoud S, Casabianca A. Psychoactive drug use among medical doctors is higher than in the general population. *Soc Sci Med.* 1991;33:269-274.
5. Webster TA. Problems of drug addiction and alcoholism among physicians. In: Scheiber SC, Doyle BB, eds. *The Impaired Physician.* New York, NY: Plenum; 1983:27-38.
6. Hughes PH, Brandenburg N, Baldwin DC, et al. Prevalence of substance use among US physicians. *JAMA.* 1992;268:2518.
7. Coombs RH. *Drug-Impaired Professionals.* Cambridge, Mass: Harvard University Press; 1997.
8. Arnetz BB, Horte L, Hedberg A. Suicide patterns among physicians related to other academics as well as to the general population. *Acta Psychiatr Scand.* 1987;75:139-143.
9. Heim E. Job stressors and coping in health professions. *Psychother Psychosom.* 1991;55:90-99.
10. Sotile WM, Sotile MO. *Beat Stress Together: The BEST Way to a Passionate Marriage, a Healthy Family, and a Productive Life.* New York, NY: John Wiley & Sons; 1999.
11. Kobasa SC, Maddi SR, Kahn S. Hardiness and health: a prospective study. *J Pers Soc Psychol.* 1982;42:707-717.
12. Miles JE, Krell R, Lin T-Y. The doctor's wife: mental illness and marital pattern. *Int J Psychiatry Med.* 1975;64:481-487.

13. Sheehan B, Sheehan DV, Whit K, Leibowitz A, Baldwin DC. A pilot study of medical student abuse: student perceptions of mistreatment and misconduct in medical school. *JAMA*. 1990;263:533-537.

14. Silver JK, Glicken AD. Medical student abuse: incidence, severity, and significance. *JAMA*. 1990;263:527-532.

15. Weisman CS, Teitelbaum MA. The work-family role system and physician productivity. *J Health Soc Behav*. 1987;28:247-257.

16. Tesch BJ, Osborne J, Simpson D, Murray SF, Spiro J. Women physicians in dual-physician relationships compared with those in other dual-career relationships. *Acad Med*. 1992;67:542-544.

17. Gabbard GO, Menninger RW. *Medical Marriages*. Washington, DC: American Psychiatric Press, Inc; 1988.

18. Olsen RD, Sande JR, Olsen GP. Maternal parenting stress in physicians' families. *Clin Pediatr*. 1991;30:586-590.

19. McCue JD. Doctors and stress: is there really a problem? *Hosp Pract*. 1986;21:7-16.

20. Schwartzberg NS, Dytell RS. Dual-earner families: the importance of work stress and family stress for psychological well-being. *Int J Occup Health Psychol*. 1999;1:211-223.

21. Bird CE. Gender, household labor, and psychological distress: the impact of the amount and division of housework. *J Health Soc Behav*. 1999;40:32-45.

Chapter 2

What Stresses Medical Marriages?

The time for the Renaissance man was the Renaissance

—Harvey MacKay, author,
   Swim With the Sharks Without Being Eaten Alive

No one enters medicine or marriage anticipating a stress-free ride. Volumes have been written about the challenges that fill each stage of medical training, medical practice, and family life. These stresses fall into three broad categories.

The Anticipated but Unavoidable

It has been said that 80 percent of the stresses we face each day are predictable. Regardless of when they marry, most medical couples are aware of certain obvious stresses in their immediate path.

- Medical school and residency will involve grueling work and study, which means that the physician will usually be exhausted and the spouse too often alone.
- Early family life will be filled with the frustration of postponing gratification—waiting until you get established to begin enjoying your life together.
- Exposure to pain, suffering, and death will take its toll on the physician.
- Once training is completed, the physician's professional life will be consumed by time pressure, financial pressure, or institutional pressure to produce.
- Fear of making mistakes may haunt a physician from the earliest days of training and throughout his or her career.

- If both spouses are physicians, multiply all of the above by two. If one of you is not, the nonphysician had better get ready to bear the brunt of the role of "stress absorber."

Even though they are clearly anticipated, these stresses are difficult to bear. But those that fall into the next two categories are the toxic ones.

The Unanticipated and Unavoidable

Many of these stresses could actually be described by saying, "We sort of anticipated this, but we had no idea it would be *this* bad." Here, too, certain dramas surface that are unique to today's medical families.

- Many medical students and residents face emotional and physical abuse.
- A backlog of debt might greet you once medical training is completed.
- There will be relentless pressure to make important decisions under urgent circumstances.
- "Physician bashing" has become the rage in recent years.
- The inflated costs of operating a medical practice will take a toll.
- The attitudes of patients toward both the physician and his or her family are often frustrating.
- Family values and the career commitments that have traditionally shaped life as a physician are incompatible.
- Many dynamic people settle into disregard for health and fitness.
- Leaving work behind at the end of the day is a never-ending difficulty.
- There is constant struggle to find the right balance in the division of roles and responsibilities within your relationship.
- Decreased autonomy in deciding how to practice medicine leads to frustration.
- Surprise! Rather than having one job, most physicians end up with at least two (and usually five) areas of career involvement: clinician, consultant, teacher, medical politician, and manager of people.
- Eventually there may be disillusionment with medicine and with your marriage.

Finally come those stresses that couples hold each other accountable for, that drain their collective energies and seem to result from choice, not happenstance.

The Anticipated and Potentially Avoidable, but Not Avoided

These are the stressors that fuel resentments and contribute to the power struggle that ruins many medical marriages. Included here are such factors as:

- Excessive ambitiousness
- Excessive materialism
- Competitiveness
- Refusal to relax and enjoy life
- Needing to control others
- Hostility and cynicism
- Constantly rushing

Controlling Yourself During Uncontrollable Times

Here we encourage you to take an honest look at what you expect from yourselves and each other. More than in earlier generations, contemporary medical couples live in a scramble. They juggle too many roles as they try to live up to unrealistic standards of excellence.

Furthermore, the "me generation" mentality of the 1960s and 1970s and the rampant materialism promoted in the 1980s combined to create the confusing 1990s. At the core of this confusion is the way that these influences from the prior three decades have affected our evaluations of the state of our relationships. We seem to have lost sight of what it means to be happy, contented, satisfied, growing, or thriving.

As we move into the twenty-first century, we are deluged with encouragement to negotiate, demand, or otherwise maneuver satisfaction of our needs within the arenas of family, work, self, and marriage.

The myth of the balanced life suggests that satisfaction in all these arenas is not only important, but also deserved and attainable. The modern ethic revolves around the assumption that such satisfaction will come your way if you try hard enough—and if the *other* people in your life could just face up to dealing with their problems and learn to be more responsible. (Here "responsible" is defined as "being more *responsive* to *my* needs.")

Many of the medical couples we have known bordered on being obsessed with self-focused quests for ever-increasing levels of satisfaction. They've wanted more appreciation from their families and more satisfaction, fulfillment, and monetary rewards from their work. They've wanted more sexual fulfillment and intimacy in their marriage, more possessions, and more time for self-focused interests. We have called the "balanced life" the Beaver Cleaver myth of the 1990s: an unrealistic yardstick that couples use to evaluate themselves. Getting lost in the quest to create this mythical balance can result in what we term the *supercouple syndrome,* in which the strategies you use to cope with your big life begin to erode caring connections with the very people for whom you are trying so hard to care.

The scramble to measure up to your own or to each other's standards of excellence has several effects, some good, some bad. It magnifies your lifestyle and forges new levels of coping strength. But it also depletes your energy—the same energy that is needed to enjoy the lifestyle that gets constructed in the process. Your very attempts to find meaning amid this scramble can hurt your intimate relationships.

Let's look at some of the complexities that face medical couples within each of these arenas.

Family

The famous family therapist Virginia Satir reminded us that, regardless of age or the stage of family life, marital partners are the architects of family systems.[1] The tone of our family life is set by our marital teamwork and our individual and collective stress levels.

Contemporary medical couples are plagued with confusing mixed messages. These messages come both from within and from outside the family. According to popular thinking, for example, both men and women are becoming more egalitarian both at work and at home. This means that men are supposedly more involved in parenting and domestic responsibilities, leaving women relatively free to exercise more choice about balancing their own roles within and outside of the family. But statistics paint a confusing picture about how couples are actually responding to these influences.

What's Really Going On. Now, as always, women are overburdened with responsibilities for home and family, and men are still struggling to find a comfortable place within their own families.

Having to or wanting to work outside the home adds complexity to the lives of contemporary women and their families. In 1980, only 38 percent of American mothers with infants worked outside the home. This figure rose to 54 percent as of 1992. As of 1995, more than 65 percent of mothers of school-aged children in America were employed outside the home.[2] And medical couples are not exceptions to these contemporary norms. By some estimates, more than 80 percent of physicians' wives work outside their homes.[3]

What about female physicians? Are their lives complicated in similar ways? The answer is yes. Through all stages of their careers, women physicians point to support and active participation from their husbands in home and family life as being *the* single most important factor—and, especially for physician-mothers, a relatively rare occurrence—in managing the stress of multiple roles. As mentioned earlier, even in dual-physician marriages, women still assume an overwhelming amount of responsibility for running the family. Women physicians, like most contemporary women, simply have added career demands to their already burgeoning responsibilities as caretakers.

Fact: Within ten years of qualification, 85 percent of married female physicians have children.[4]

Fact: When physician mothers opt to continue in medicine, they work the same number of hours as their childless women-physician peers.[5]

Fact: When they are employed full-time, female physicians continue to assume almost full-time responsibility for running their home and family life.[6]

Fact: Most women physicians work full-time, if not immediately, then eventually. A woman physician practices an average of twenty-four years of full-time equivalent during her medical career.[7]

What's going on here? Why are contemporary women overburdened with so many roles? Some researchers suggest that the overburdening is primarily due to male avoidance of involvement in family life.[8]

Although women have flooded the workplace—and doubled their own stress loads—over the past twenty years, pollsters have found that, as recently as the early 1990s, men's average time performing household tasks has increased only 6 percent during this same period.[9]

But this picture is changing.

What About Men?   From the facts mentioned above, it seems that, for the most part, men are still stuck in their overlearned habit of avoiding too much involvement with loved ones by "operating" in the outside world. But a growing body of evidence suggests that, taken alone, these facts don't really paint a complete picture of contemporary families. These days, men, too, are struggling to find balance in their multiple roles. Arguably, while women still do more work *inside* the home per week than men, men spend more *total* time working in their multiple roles than do women.[10]

In his provocative book *Women Can't Hear What Men Don't Say*,[11] psychologist Warren Farrell points out that such facts do not reflect a *new* phenomenon.

Fact: A 1975 nationwide sampling of households found that, when all child care, housework, work outside the home, commuting, and gardening were added together, husbands did 53 percent of the total work; wives, 47 percent.[12]

Recent years have evidenced a booming interest in masculine psychology. One of its most important messages is that it is time for men to end the legacy of father-absent families. Perhaps due to such influences, men have joined women in the ranks of achievers who are deeply concerned about the competing demands of home and work.

Fact: A 1979 survey found that only 12 percent of men indicated that they felt stressed by the struggle to balance home and work responsibilities. When this survey was repeated in 1989, the percentage of men reporting such stress had soared to 72 percent.[9]

Fact: Conflict about not having enough time to spend with their families or with their spouses alone is *the most frequent complaint* of male physicians.[13-15]

Fact: Research with professional groups such as physicians and attorneys has repeatedly documented that between 30 and 54 percent of those surveyed wish to change careers in hopes of creating a more comfortable work-family balance.[16,17]

More men than ever are saying they want increased hands-on involvement in their family lives. However, it seems that by and large male physicians are still filling their lives with tasks, chores, and challenges that take them away from their family relationships. In the privacy of our counseling sessions, most men admit feeling anxiety about spending much of their time or energy actually doing things *with their families.*

Fact: When male physicians become parents, they *increase* their hours at work.[5]

More men than ever before are reporting inner conflict about the work-family balance in their life, yet are still spending their best energy *outside* their family relationships. Why is this? Ostensibly, it is due to increased pressures that come from the financial demands of raising a family and the strong probability that once a couple has children, it will be the wife who stops working in order to focus on parenting. But there are two other perspectives that are worth considering here. According to Jerrold Lee Shapiro, author of *The Measure of A Man: Becoming the Father You Wish Your Father Had Been,* men don't absent themselves from active participation in family life out of some self-centered decision to avoid changing dirty diapers; instead, they are *excluded* from positions of power and responsibility within their domestic lives.[18] Shapiro claims that many wives are reluctant to truly share family and domestic control and responsibility with their husbands. Men who do focus on parenting and running their households often find themselves relegated to the status of a second-rate mother rather than first-rate father.

Recent research regarding what has been termed the "maternal gatekeeping" phenomenon supports Shapiro's claim.[19] Maternal gatekeeping happens when a working mother who also holds traditional conceptualizations of family roles shows reluctance to relinquish responsibility for family matters by setting rigid, demanding standards of excellence to which she holds herself and her mate accountable. According to Brigham Young University Family Studies Center researchers Sarah Allen and Alan Hawkins, "gatekeepers" discourage their husbands' involvement by redoing tasks, criticizing, creating unbending standards, or demeaning efforts to share domestic responsibilities.[19] These wives protect their domestic role by acting as household managers who organize, delegate, plan, schedule, and oversee the work done by their husbands. Doing so encourages fathers to assume the role of a "helper" who waits until asked to help and who needs explicit directions to carry out child care or domestic chores. From their recent study of 622 dual-earner couples, Allen and Hawkins found that 20 to 25 percent of mothers may be classified as "gatekeepers."[19]

Our own clinical experiences suggest that the distress experienced by male physicians when they spend extended time with their loved ones may have multiple origins. For some, this stress may come from a lack of nurturing skills or the sadness that is engendered when parenting reminds a man that *he* was not nurtured by his own father. Certain men also find it difficult to turn off high-powered coping mechanisms and simply connect with loved ones.

One point seems obvious: Among contemporary medical couples, *both* sexes are burdened with too many roles and responsibilities.

Wellesley College psychologist Rosalind Barnett and colleagues studied 300 dual-career couples and found that job stresses have an equal effect on men's and women's mental health; most interestingly, no differences existed in the importance of family to married men and women.[20]

The stresses facing medical families are not limited to marital struggles over shared responsibilities. Families today are bombarded with abnormal pressures to consume goods, stimulate children, and hold together in the face of social influences that threaten to splinter family structure and unity. In addition, the escalating costs of such essentials as medical care, education, and maintaining a household, coupled with the diminished value of the dollar, create enormous pressures.

Work

This takes us to the next element being juggled by today's medical couples: work. The new work ethic in our culture mixes a willingness and necessity to work hard to achieve our goals with a narcissistic expectation that these goals will be met. This struggle is especially evident in dual-career couples, but it also occurs in families with only one wage earner.

A 1993 *Time* magazine article[9] pointed out the mixed messages given in the contemporary workplace regarding the value placed on family life. The article made the point that career advancement in corporate America is seriously hindered when men prioritize their family life over the hard-driving, self-sacrificing work ethic. A 1989 survey of medium and large private employers found that only 1 percent of employees had the option of paid paternity leave and just 18 percent could take unpaid paternity leave.[9] Even when such leave was available, only about 7 percent of men working in large corporations took advantage of it.[9]

To our knowledge, the notion of paid paternity leave has not yet pene-trated the medical world. In truth, the opposite ethic still prevails in most medical settings. A physician on the faculty of a major teaching hospital, the father of five young children, recently reported to us that although he typically works seventy hours per week and is gaining a national reputa-tion in his field, he is regularly admonished to "begin choosing your career over your family if you expect to advance in this department."

Perhaps this is why, despite modern-day messages proclaiming a woman's right to her own career, most medical marriages revolve around the career of the physician-husband. This is obvious in the case of a tradi-tional medical marriage: A busy physician marries a loving and nurturing wife who cooperates with him in creating a life that facilitates his career, and the couple become a living example of what has been termed a "two-person career."

But even dual-physician marriages often depend on a traditional mari-tal arrangement that allows the husband to devote his time and energy to work. This often means that the physician-wife defers to the career needs of her physician-husband when choosing a specialty, deciding how much to work, or deciding whether to disrupt her own career in order to relocate for her husband-physician's career.

Within corporate America it may be unwise for women to take preg-nancy leave. In *Women and the Work/Family Dilemma*, Deborah Swiss and Judith Walker summarized the responses of 902 female graduates of Harvard's law, medical, and business schools, and noted that in some instances professional women attempted to avoid career setbacks by giv-ing birth to their babies on Friday and returning to work on Monday![21] A number of researchers have documented that upwards of 40 percent of female physicians are subjected to scorn and discrimination from both col-leagues and superiors if they become pregnant.[22,23] In fact, as of the late 1980s, only 32 percent of teaching hospitals had formal maternity leave policies.[24,25]

The Clashing Generations

Now more than ever, both men and women are in conflict about their home and work roles. The desire of younger people to have lives that do not revolve exclusively around work often leads to clashes with the older generation of professionals. A senior partner in a large group medical prac-tice recently lamented to us:

What is wrong with this new crop of physicians? We recruit only the top 10 percent of graduating classes from outstanding medical schools. These physicians show up for work expecting six to eight weeks of vaca-tion, time off for their kids' ball games, a limited number of nights on call, and all kinds of things that I didn't get until I had been in practice for fifteen years, if at all! Of course, they also want to make good money, even though they claim that they aren't that interested in money. What is the deal with these people!

For the most part, contemporary young couples do not want to be like the previous generation; they want a more comfortable balance among work, family, romance, and self-interests, and they claim they are willing to trade money for a balanced lifestyle. As stated by Michael Myers in his thoughtful book *Doctors' Marriages: A Look at the Problems and Their Solutions:*

> Younger physicians as a rule are determined not to make medicine their whole raison d'être. They approach their work as diligently as their elders, but with a different perspective. Most accept the fact that the traditional medical marriage is becoming largely historical and that they have many other responsibilities besides their patients. And fortunately, I think that physicians are beginning to feel less guilty about working fewer hours per week and taking well-earned or overdue vacations."[26]

We sincerely hope that this last statement proves to be true. Unfortunately, the facts suggest that while physicians are struggling to increase their attention to at-home responsibilities, they are continuing to work longer and harder than most other professionals.

Fact: Three times as many physicians as other professionals spend sixty hours or more a week on the job, working in a profession that most researchers suggest is more stressful than many.[27]

The most frequent stresses cited by physicians and their loved ones are diminished leisure time and the struggle to balance time spent in career versus family pursuits. Surveys consistently find that male physicians work, on average, sixty to eighty hours per week, with approximately 38 percent reporting that they work over eighty hours per week.[28] Recent surveys call into question whether the new work ethic is really leading to greater balance in the lives of physicians and their mates. On the pessimistic side is a report[28] on 217 academic surgeons (only eight were female) and 165 of their spouses that indicated that one fourth of the couples spent fewer than two hours each week alone with each other. In this survey, 48 percent of the physicians' spouses were employed outside the home, and one-third of these nonphysician spouses (all but eight of whom were women) reported spending fewer than six hours each week with their families. Furthermore, this survey found that, although these surgeons were entitled to an average of four or more weeks of vacation each year, 70 percent actually used only three or less.

Another study[29] monitored a medical couple during the course of a week and found that, on average, the physician-father spent four minutes a day with his son as his primary focus of attention and only thirty-eight minutes a day in general contact with the child.

In contrast, recent time diary data from a nationally representative sample of 1,761 children up to twelve years of age who lived with both their parents in 1997 reported that, on average, fathers spend 2.5 hours each weekday and 6.2 hours a day on weekends attending to their children.[30,31]

It seems that both the physicians *and* the nonphysicians in modern-day medical marriages are espousing a new work ethic but may be living in an ever-tightening time crunch. This crunch is fueled by expanded expectations within a third arena of life—self-actualization.

Self

Prior generations concentrated less than the current one on how much money they had, how they looked, and to what extent their lives entertained and fulfilled them. Whereas they valued working hard, surviving, and doing the "right" things, more recent generations bring into their marriages a new and expanded set of values that center on self-interests.

Referring to research by the Public Agenda Foundation and the Aspen Institute for Humanistic Studies, author Perry Pascarella observed:

> These new values emphasize personal creativity, self-expression, adventure, the enjoyment of living for its own sake, the savoring of personal relationships, harmony with nature, the search for the sacred, and the satisfaction that comes with exploring the full richness of human experience.[32]

Many contemporary social researchers have confirmed the predictions Pascarella expressed in his 1984 book *The New Achievers: Creating a Modern Work Ethic*:

> We can see around us today people grasping for ways to build a wholeness of self and to find a place in some greater unity. . . . Perhaps at no time in man's history have people been so insistent on pursuing their search for meaning and significance. We are moving toward a "self-realization ethic," says futurist Willis Harman. We are beginning to fashion a "self-development ethic," says psychoanalyst Michael Maccoby. And after studying the results of many surveys—his own and others'—of American attitudes and values, social analyst Daniel Yankelovich suspects we are moving toward an "ethic of commitment." These analysts, too, are saying that people are trying to break through the tight definition that has been imposed on them. People are turning inward, reaching outward, and looking upward. The drive toward personal growth leads many to commit to things outside themselves.[32]

We do not believe that this increased self-absorption is all bad. We counsel many physicians and their hard-driving mates who mourn how little they have relaxed or played during the course of their lives to carve out time for regular "recess." In fact, we coach many couples to do so as a means of renewing their energy and preserving their health.

Unfortunately, many of them cooperate in creating and perpetuating a way of life that diminishes their primary protection against burnout—caring connection with the people around them. Often, their drive toward personal growth leads them to commit to things outside of themselves, and they create stress-filled lives. Then they suffer from the wear and tear of keeping up with what they have created. They then urgently (and sometimes angrily) declare their right to be individualistic, sometimes to inappropriate degrees.[33]

Marriage

The final ball that contemporary couples juggle—along with commitments to family, work, and self—is marriage. These days, we demand and expect (of ourselves and of each other) tolerance, nurturing, and passion as we go about the business of keeping up with the other three arenas deemed essential to having it all. Here we offer a quote from psychologist and author Marion Solomon to highlight the marital dilemma that is often caused by our lofty expectations:

> We have been raised to expect that our lives can be busy, exciting, fulfilling, and materially successful. We believe that marriage should be part of that. . . . In the idealized image of the modern American couple . . . it is assumed that members of both sexes can "have it all"—a successful career and a happy family life. In the fantasy, everyone gets what he or she wants. But that is not what most men and women experience. Both men and women have lost the clear knowledge of what is expected of them, individually and in relationships. We are bombarded with a series of cultural myths that tell us that we can have it all, that we must be responsible to ourselves first, that a successful life depends more on financial success than on ethical or moral values. The myths of relationships permeate our lives with narcissistic expectations.[33]

What Do You Value?

The first step in determining whether, where, and how these multiple roles and multiple expectations create stress in your life and in your marriage is identifying your respective value systems. Take a minute to complete the following exercise.

Values Inventory

Each of you should complete the first part of this exercise *solo*, not as a couple. Look over the following list of values. If you had to choose to have only five of these things in your life, which would you choose? Answer according to what *you* truly value, not what you think you *should* value, or what your *spouse* values. Rank the five factors in order of importance.*

Security	Status	Recognition
Fame	Being liked	Belonging
Approval	Affection	Spirituality
Adventure	Fun	Friendships
Acceptance	Power	Service
Achievement	Authority	Physical health
Glamor	Money	Relaxation
Sexual fun	Family ties	Parenting
Passion	Learning	Culture

*Obviously, this list is not exhaustive, and entries are not mutually exclusive. We offer this exercise merely to stimulate your thinking and your discussion. Add to it as needed to clarify your personal values.

Next, share your respective lists of values. Note where you agree and disagree; how are you similar and different? Explain the importance of the values you checked. Discuss the *extent* to which your values vary. Notice where you strongly differ (e.g., perhaps one of you highly values sexual fun, and the other has no interest in sex). Also note the extent to which your collective values spread across the four arenas mentioned above: family, work, self, and marriage.

While bearing in mind the breadth of your collective values, consider another fact. Despite the ever-expanding scope of our wants and needs, our lives continue to be constrained by the great equalizer expressed in the following equation: $7 \times 24 = 168$.

Now, as always, the week continues to consist of seven twenty-four-hour days. The roles and demands that we place on ourselves and each other have expanded, but the actual time we have for these things has remained the same.

In his book *Successful Time Management: A Self-Teaching Guide*, time management expert Jack Ferner points out a sobering fact. Once you subtract from this 168 hours the amount of time spent each week eating, sleeping, working outside your home for forty to fifty hours (which, we know, means a "light workweek" for some of you), and the time spent attending to chores, what will remain for most people is approximately thirty-five hours per week.[34] That means that, other than work and responsibilities, most of us have as few as thirty-five hours per week to do *all* else that will define what and who we are in this life!

Discussing the stresses that face physicians, Joseph Trainer put it this way:

Sleep 49 hours; work 60 hours; study groups and medical meetings 6 hours; civic, non-medical activities 2 hours; meal times (some at home) 14 hours; emergencies 10 hours; hobbies or exercise 7 hours. This leaves 20 hours in the week to go to the toilet, get the car serviced, do some essential shopping, handle business matters. If the physician is unusually effective, he may find 6 hours a week for the company of his wife, and if he has 2 children, each will come in for 3 hours apiece. For someone living in the upper echelon of society, able to come and go far better than most of his fellow citizens, this does not read like a luxurious life, nor does it carry much weight as family life.[35]

Redefining Balance

Of *your* discretionary hours last week, how many were spent actually engaging in some activity that matched your primary values? For example, if you checked "family ties" or "learning" or "passion" on the values inventory, what did you actually *do* last week to give expression to this value? Furthermore, what did you do to help your partner accomplish something within each of his or her primary values?

Remember: this is *your* life and *your* marriage. These are *your* values. A hidden stress in the lives of many high-powered people is that they do not live in harmony with their inner values. Physician Jack McCue cautioned his colleagues that if the answer to the question "What would you like to be doing ten years from now?" is not "What I am doing now," then it was time for a serious self-examination and redesigning of one's life.

For most people this redesign involves creating a new kind of balance among family, work, self, and marriage. For both situational and psychological reasons, this is an inherently difficult task for physicians.

Fact: Research in Sweden has shown that over one fourth of physicians have difficulty winding down following a regular workday, and that over 30 percent of physicians (compared to only 10 percent of other professionals) report regularly being too tired to engage in social activities, to meet friends, and to interact with family following a regular workday.[36]

How can you create perfect balance when overinvolvement in one of the four arenas uses up the vast majority of your time and energy? The answer is simple: You can't. In fact, we misconstrue the term "balance." Remember that balance is dynamic, not a static process. The key is repeatedly and regularly to readjust your efforts and attend to the arenas of your life that have been relatively neglected in the immediate past. But it *is* possible to create a *reasonable* degree of balance across these arenas within any reasonable chunk of time, such as a week or a month. It is virtually impossible to have a sense of well-being without this balance. Overfocusing in one area to the exclusion of others will hurt your life. Put another way, this "reasonable balance" is essential if you are to move out of the "wait until" and into the "here and now" in your marriage.

References

1. Satir V. *Conjoint Family Therapy*. Palo Alto, Calif: Science and Behavior Books; 1964.
2. Barnett RC, Rivers C. *She Works/He Works: How Two-Income Families are Happier, Healthier, and Better Off*. San Francisco, Calif: Harper; 1996.
3. Moore EE. Presidential address: swimming with the sharks—without the family being eaten alive. *Surgery*. 1990;108:125-138.
4. Stephen PJ. Career patterns of women medical graduates, 1974-1984. *Med Educ*. 1987;21:255-259.
5. Mitchell JB. Why do women physicians work fewer hours than men physicians? *Inquiry*. 1984;21:361-368.
6. Tesch BJ, Osborne J, Simpson D, Murray SF, Spiro J. Women physicians in dual-physician relationships compared with those in other dual-career relationships. *Acad Med*. 1992;67:542-544.
7. Swerdlow AJ, McNeilly RH, Rue ER. Women doctors in training: problems and progress. *Br Med J*. 1980;281:754-758.
8. Zick CD, McCullough JL. Trends in married couples' time use: evidence from 1977-1978 and 1987-1988. *Sex Roles*. 1991;24:459-487.
9. Gibbs NR. Bringing up father. *Time*. June 28, 1993:53-56.
10. Juster FT, Stafford FP. The allocation of time: empirical findings, behavioral models, and problems of measurement. *J Econ Literature*. 1991;292:477.
11. Farrell W. *Women Can't Hear What Men Don't Say: Destroying Myths, Creating Love*. New York, NY: Jeremy P. Tarcher/Putnam; 1999.
12. Hill M. Patterns of time use. In: Juster FT, Stafford FP, eds. *Time, Goods, and Well-Being*. Ann Arbor: Institute for Social Research, University of Michigan; 1985.
13. Ahern M. Survey of Florida physicians: characteristics and satisfaction. *J Fla Med Assoc*. 1993;80:752-757.
14. Graham J, Ramirez AJ, Cull A, Finlay I, Hoy A, Richards MA. Job stress and satisfaction among palliative physicians. *Palliative Med*. 1996;10:185-194.
15. Kam K. Finding balance: if not now, when? *Hippocrates*. 1998;12:38-45.
16. Dayton M. Survey: one in five suffering from stress. *Lawyers Monthly*. 1991;3:1-5.
17. McCue J. Doctors and stress: is there really a problem? *Hosp Pract*. 1986;21:7-16.
18. Shapiro JL. *The Measure of a Man: Becoming the Father You Wish Your Father Had Been*. Berkley,Calif: Berkley Publishing Group; 1995.
19. Allen SM, Hawkins AJ. Maternal gatekeeping: mothers' beliefs and behaviors that inhibit greater father involvement in family work. *J Marriage Fam*. 1999;61:199-212.
20. Cited in: Adler T. Stress from work, home hits men, women equally. *APA Monitor*. 1993;247:11-14.
21. Swiss D, Walker J. *Women and the Work/Family Dilemma: How Today's Professional Women Are Confronting the Maternal Wall*. New York, NY: John Wiley & Sons, Inc; 1993.

22. Lenhart SA. Physician mothers: a conceptual model for planning and coping with motherhood and medical practice. *JAMA*. 1992;47:87-93.

23. Sayres M, Wyshak G, Denterlein G, et al. Pregnanacy during residency. *N Engl J Med* 1986;314:418-423.

24. Tech J. A look at maternity leave spolicies in COTH hospitals. In: *COTH Report, Special Supplement*. Washington, DC: Association of American Medical Schools; 1987.

25. Silva BM. Pregnancy during residency: a look at the issues. *JAMA*. 1992;47:71-75.

26. Myers M. *Doctors' Marriages: A Look at the Problems and Their Solutions*. New York, NY: Plenum Medical Book Co; 1988:223.

27. Gross EB. Gender differences in physician stress. *JAMA*. 1992;47:107-114.

28. Fabri PJ, McDaniel MD, Gaskill HV, et al. Great expectations: stress and the medical family. *J Surg Res*. 1989;47:379-382.

29. Gerber LA. *Married to Their Careers: Family Dilemmas in Doctors' Lives*. New York, NY: Tavistock; 1983.

30. Yeung WJ. Multiple domains of paternal involvement. Paper presented at: Annual Meeting for Population Association of America; 1999; New York, NY.

31. Yeung WJ, Sandberg J, Davis-Kean P, Hofferth S. Children's time-use with fathers in intact families. Paper presented at: Annual Meeting for Population Association of America; 1998; Chicago, Ill.

32. Pascarella P. *The New Achievers: Creating a Modern Work Ethic*. New York, NY: The Free Press; 1984:88.

33. Solomon M. *Narcissism and Intimacy: Love and Marriage in an Age of Confusion*. New York, NY: WW Norton; 1989:9.

34. Ferner J. *Successful Time Management: A Self-Teaching Guide*. New York, NY: John Wiley & Sons, Inc; 1980.

35. Trainer JB. Is the medical marriage hazardous to your health? *J Fla Med Assoc*. 1981;68:261-264.

36. Arnetz BB. White collar stress: what studies of physicians can teach us. *Psychother Psychosom*. 1991;55:197-200.

Chapter 3

Personality and Coping

Human beings tend to live too far within self-imposed limits.

—William James

Many physicians and their spouses are suffering. Their very attempts to solve their problems only exacerbate them. They use their collective, high-powered style of coping to acclimate to more and more stress. They learn to focus their energies and maximize their efficiency, all the while struggling against the anxiety that their progress will be impeded by others' inefficiency or opposition. They become subtly (or not so subtly) controlling in their interactions with others. The habit of doing and thinking more than one thing at once interferes with their ability to connect with others. They forget how to relax and play. They begin to confuse relief with pleasure. Struggling becomes a way of life even when there is no reason to struggle.

It is difficult to avoid this trap. As you face unrelenting stress of any sort—including that which results from working as a physician or living with one—you will automatically reach for "ace in the hole" coping strategies, those ways of calming inner tensions that seem most familiar. Like most people, you will lock in these coping strategies, even if they are not generating the outcomes you want. Especially when facing relationship tensions, it is human nature to try harder to make a certain coping strategy work rather than to try something new and different.

Several facts support our observation that physicians and their loved ones are at particular risk of suffering this misguided coping syndrome.

Fact: Between 30 and 50 percent of physicians report anxiety, sleeplessness, or depression in reaction to personal problems—percentages that are significantly higher than in other professions.[1-3]

Fact: Despite the aforementioned documented tendencies to over-work and then have difficulty winding down, approximately 30 per-cent of physicians attempt to relax after work by simply switching to another form of toil—working around the house.[3]

Fact: While the suicide rate for physicians is two times that of the general population, it is also true that the rate of suicide is greater for physicians' wives than for wives of any other professional group.[4,5]

Can these phenomena simply be attributed to the high levels of stress associated with the practice of medicine? We think not. The sociological literature has repeatedly pointed out that such extrinsic factors as work-related stress play a less important role in determining overall well-being than do such factors as emotional support from each other and general psychosocial background. It is unlikely that the stresses inherent in medical marriage can, in and of themselves, wreak this degree of havoc in your personal adjustment. Another possible explanation is that certain people are predisposed to crumble under the pressures that attend a medical marriage.

A famous longitudinal study of physicians conducted by George Vaillant and colleagues[6] supports this notion. They found that the physicians who become casualties of the rigors of medical training and practice are those who *enter* the profession suffering from fundamental insecurities—low self-esteem, emotional dependency, social anxiety, and a tendency toward depression. This finding has been replicated in subsequent studies that have suggested that approximately 40 percent of those physicians who committed suicide brought symptoms of emotional and psychological problems with them into medical training; 60 percent became symptomatic in reaction to the stresses and strains of medical education and practice.[7]

In a similar vein, the plight of overstressed wives of physicians has been depicted simplistically as the *result* of the pressures that come with being married to a physician. Evaluations of small numbers of psychiatrically hospitalized women have led to the notion that physicians' wives tend to be overly dependent, angry, depressive, prone to substance abuse and somatization disorder, and unhappily married. What is often misrepresented—or blatantly omitted—in discussions of this topic is that the people on whom this stereotyping is based were hospitalized women, the majority of whom were from families that had histories of emotional and psychiatric disturbances. It would be more appropriate to interpret the results of these studies as indicating that the physician-spouses who become most disturbed in the course of a medical marriage may be those who *enter* the marriage predisposed to struggle. As Vaillant commented, many physicians seem to have "painful and unstable marriages because they married not partners but patients."[6]

What Do Physicians and Their Spouses Bring Into Marriage?

This, of course, is a question that is impossible to answer. It always amazes us when researchers provide definitive thoughts on the "typical physician personality" or the "typical spouse of a physician." Only someone who "studies" medical couples (rather than listening to their struggles and getting to know them) would presume to make sweeping statements about such a diverse population. With this caveat registered, we present the following brief overview of the research as a way of setting the stage for what we believe to be a more sensible (and more humane) way of understanding each other.

For the most part, research in this area has focused on physicians, not their spouses. The most often quoted investigations have proposed that, as a group, physicians' personality characteristics tend to be homogeneous. It has been suggested that, starting in childhood, many physicians spend a lifetime struggling. Physicians often report that they became attracted to medicine as a profession at an early age. A number of studies of the early life experiences of physicians have examined the question of why a child would be compelled to idealize a profession as demanding as medicine. It seems that "for some physicians the aspiration to be a physician is part and parcel of the same personality traits which lead him to make an unsatisfactory marriage."[8]

As was mentioned previously, physicians tend to describe their childhoods as lacking in emotional nurturing from parental figures. The result? From a young age, many learn to repress awareness of their own needs and feelings and to delay gratification as they steadily work at gaining approval.

This quest to gain approval pervades the life cycle of these physicians and is supposedly fueled by chronically low self-esteem, which is said to perpetuate one of two behaviors.

Some of these physicians suffer from a relentless and tormenting drive to present an inflated persona to the world. They may become so preoccupied with their own frustrated needs and wants that they appear to be pathologically narcissistic, a condition in which a fragile sense of self is defended by dealing with the world in a manner that suggests that one is all-important and omnipotent.

For other physicians, the chronic struggle to soothe a damaged sense of self and to gain some modicum of fulfillment leads to an effort to be all things to all people. Here the original desire for an intimate and loving relationship with a nurturing parent is replaced with an endless quest to gain respect from colleagues and community. Becoming a caretaker *par excellence* creates the opportunity to give to others what was never received as a child.

For many physicians, the need to be admired and appreciated in order to compensate for childhood narcissistic injuries leads to workaholism. These psychological factors, coupled with the relentless demands of medical education and practice, result in what are supposedly the hallmark psychological characteristics of physicians:

- Compulsiveness
- Perfectionism
- Insistence that others submit to their way of doing things
- Emotional detachment
- Workaholism
- Loss of playfulness
- Poor interpersonal relationships
- The "neurotic triad of doubt, guilt, and an exaggerated sense of responsibility"[3,9]

Indeed, it does appear that physicians, more than other professionals, are likely to display such personality and coping characteristics. Most importantly, it appears that these same psychological characteristics compel many physicians to choreograph a stress-generating two-step throughout their lives. First, they fill their lives with excessive work demands and pressures; then they cope with work stress in ways that compound their struggles. While 46 percent of a sample of 50 lawyers indicated that they respond to periods of excessive work pressure by taking time off to recuperate, 50 percent of a comparable sample of 100 physicians indicated that they respond to periods of increased work pressure by *increasing* their time spent at work.[10] Perhaps this explains another observation: For physicians (as compared to lawyers), the ratio of the incidence of depression as a result of personal stress is three to one.[10]

Such data bear out the frequently stated notion that

Qualities that make for excellence in the physician (ie, dedication to the pursuit of knowledge, commitment to patients, attention to detail, thoroughness, willingness to work hard for long periods of time) may be so demanding and absorbing that the needs of the physician's family members may be neglected.[11]

While interesting and no doubt helpful to many people, this literature is too general and pejorative in its descriptions of physicians. Not captured here are the factors that create varying coping patterns—positive and negative—that fill the private lives of physicians and their loved ones.

Understanding Personality

Mental health professionals often needlessly complicate the issue of personality. While it is true that many people struggle with complex psychological problems, most of us are driven by rather simple psychological factors:

- We all have inner fears and insecurities.
- We learn how to cope based on what works best during crucial times of our life.
- In coping with stress, we do the best we can, given what we know about how to avoid pain or attain pleasure.
- Each of us is capable of learning new ways of coping.
- However, our old coping patterns feel like our safest bets; these are the strategies that we automatically reach for during stressful times.
- Unfortunately, old coping habits sometimes exacerbate rather than eliminate stress.

What worked in helping us cope in the past may not work so well in dealing with current stresses.

Personality Drivers

A simple yet useful way of thinking about personality and coping is called *transactional analysis*, which in part proposes that most of us develop combinations of six ways of driving ourselves as we organize our coping efforts. These coping patterns are called *drivers* because, during stressful times, we seem to be driven to act in ways that correspond with one or more of these themes. These coping mechanisms drive our ways of thinking, behaving, and feeling and are crucial in shaping both our stress reactions and our relationships.

Being Strong. If you were taught that your role in life is to be stoic, never complaining about your pains and fears, you probably are driven by a *Being Strong* personality theme. You are likely to have trouble asking for support and help during hard times. You may even have trouble noticing when you need help, because you tend to numb yourself to feelings of vulnerability and fear. Instead, you are probably in the habit of paying attention to more "powerful" feelings, such as anger. The result can be lonely and numbing as you go through life blunting your emotional awareness.

Being Perfect. If you drive yourself with a *Being Perfect* personality theme, you are probably accustomed to feeling anxious, irritable, and guilty. Because perfection is impossible to attain, you spend much of your time fussing—at yourself for your own blemishes, and at others for their shortcomings.

Trying Hard. Some of us learn to equate self-worth with fatigue. We have been taught that our value lies in our ability to struggle longer and harder than others. If you are driven by a *Trying Hard* personality, you may have difficulty determining when you have worked hard enough to deserve a rest, and you probably feel anxious when you try to relax or play. When caught in *Trying Hard*, you deal with stress by narrowly focusing on the tasks at hand, relentlessly pursuing your goals and only resting once your fatigue builds to exhaustion.

Pleasing Others. If you have difficulty being appropriately self-focused and self-nurturing without feeling guilty, then you are probably driven by a *Pleasing Others* personality. Such individuals have difficulty determining when it is okay to say "no" to requests from others and difficulty figuring out their own needs and wants. Even when you *are* aware of your needs and wants, you probably have difficulty asking for your fair share of love and attention. In this self-sacrificing way of living, you may become regularly exhausted by your relationships and experience brief periods of withdrawal and depression as an indirect way of gaining relief. Unfortunately, these periods of withdrawal tend to fuel guilt and anxiety, which may catapult you back into a *Pleasing Others* flurry.

Hurrying. Some of us were taught to rush through life. If you are driven by a *Hurrying* personality, you probably live with an internal sense of urgency about a reality that faces us all: there is more to do than time allows. When forced to slow down (by health problems, the "slowness" of others, or your own limitations), you are likely to suffer anxiety, frustration, and irritability.

Being Careful. If you often feel free-floating anxiety—scared and anxious but unaware of what is bothering you—you probably learned to cope with life by *Being Careful*. You may obsessively worry as you react to changes in your life. You are probably a real pro at anticipating what might go wrong even when all is going well. Obsessed with this innate tendency to conjure up catastrophic visions, those driven by *Being Careful* are likely to experience high anxiety when faced with decisions. Some focus their worry on the potential consequences of their own decisions. Others worry about decisions made by loved ones. The worst-case scenarios that fill their imagination begin to *feel* like realities. In this way, these people plague themselves (and their loved ones) with their paralyzing fear of change.

Coping Patterns and Pitfalls

You probably use all of these coping patterns to different degrees at different times. Indeed, each of them can be helpful; each works sometimes. But if you lock into your most familiar driver, you limit your flexibility and become stuck in a rigid way of coping. Any overused coping strategy also leaves you feeling one version or another of pain. There are various signs that your coping efforts are not working.

Signs of Personality-based Stress

If you cope rigidly by:	then your stress symptom is likely to be:
Being strong	Loneliness and numbness
Trying hard	Fatigue and joylessness
Pleasing others	Guilt, anxiety, and withdrawal
Being perfect	Guilt, irritability, and obsessing
Being careful	Fear and difficulty making decisions
Hurrying	Anxiety and urgency

Looking over the above list, you can see that symptoms of coping with stress vary, depending on your personality makeup. Different people know they are stressed when they feel numb, fatigued, withdrawn, irritated, or afraid. This is an important point, especially for those who discount the notion that stress affects them. We often make the mistake of assuming that if we are not acting like "nervous wrecks," we must not be stressed. High-powered people are often driven by personality programming that short-circuits anxiety. Accordingly, stress is more likely to be experienced as loneliness, numbness, guilt, fatigue, irritability, urgency— anything but anxiety.

Learning to Drive: Where Does This Stuff Come From?

Since the days of Sigmund Freud, various theorists have posited that personality develops from our early life experiences. Until we became parents ourselves, we, like many of our colleagues, tried to get our clients to empower themselves and change their lives by mustering up a healthy dose of anger at their parents. The unspoken motto of many psychotherapists seems to be: "The path to mental health is paved with blame of the client's parents for all that they did and did not do during his or her childhood."

Once we became parents, we changed our professional tune. We soon found ourselves joking that, rather than saving money to send our daughters, Rebecca and Julia, to college, we were actually saving to send them to psychotherapy; we knew that we were messing those kids up in some way, but we just couldn't figure out how! Now our girls are grown, and here we sit, waiting for some as-yet-undetermined therapist type to one day teach our babies how we "damaged" their precious psyches.

The role models and messages from the family you grew up in write the initial chapters of your personality script. However, the experiences of your current life—including experiences with mates, mentors, and colleagues—also have formidable personality-scripting effects. None of us copes in any singular way, and no single coping strategy works well in all arenas of life. The coping patterns that promote success at work may only serve to alienate you from your loved ones. And what you need to do in order to be loved may not be an effective way of attaining success at work. Furthermore, what worked to create harmony in the family you grew up in might not work so well with your spouse or children.

Given these caveats, examining the "old stuff" of your life is still an enlightening way to begin answering the question, "How did I get this way?"

Splitting

Much of personality development is based on an unfortunate fact of life: None of our emotional needs are ever perfectly satisfied. Based on the peculiarities of the formative influences in our lives, we each are taught to feel uncomfortable with certain ways of behaving, thinking, or feeling that otherwise would become a natural, healthy part of our behavioral and emotional repertoire. No significant figures in our life are ever perfect caretakers. They probably did the best they could in coping with their lives, including areas that had to do with caring for us. Their caretaking was shaped by their own life experiences and was limited by their insecurities. (These statements apply to everyone: our parents, other significant figures in our lives, and our mates.)

Because the people that fill our life are more comfortable responding to certain of our emotions and behaviors than others, each of us develops an internal psychological "splitting" that lurks at the core of our sense of self. One part of the split contains the characteristics that please those around us based on *their* needs, not ours. We are taught that these are admirable aspects of ourselves. We quickly learn that expressing these "good self" traits inspires a positive outcome. These behaviors, thoughts, or feelings will allow us to either gain pleasure or avoid pain.

On the other hand, any thoughts, feelings, needs, or wants that meet with disapproval, discomfort, or shaming from significant others get repressed and stored in the unexpressed or "bad" aspect of self. Because we are motivated to avoid pain and gain pleasure, we tend to fill our life with choices that further our internal splits. We overexpress our "good" traits and underexpress our "bad" ones. Accordingly, we increase our familiarity and comfort with the expressed components of ourselves, but we are left with festering, lingering doubt and discomfort about the unexpressed thoughts, feelings, and needs in ourselves. In this way, a split develops between our expressed and unexpressed selves.

If the split is extreme, personality disorders develop. People with personality disorders tend to be filled with rage that is stored in the unexpressed self—anger that masks hurts that came from abuse or neglect at the hands of narcissistic or uncaring parents.

In some families, for example, parents are so filled with their own insecurities, preoccupations, or stresses that the child is taught to assume the role of emotional caretaker for the parents. The poignant book *Drama of the Gifted Child* sheds light on the difficulties that can result. In the following passages, author Alice Miller describes the effects that mothers with unresolved narcissistic personality disturbances may have on their offspring.

> What these mothers had once failed to find in their own mothers they (are) able to find in their children: someone at their disposal who can be used as an echo, who can be controlled, is completely centered on them, will never desert them, and offers full attention and admiration. . . . Yet, what is missing above all is the framework within which the child could experience his feelings and his emotions. Instead, he develops something the mother needs, and this certainly saves his life at the time, but it nevertheless may prevent him, throughout his life, from being himself.[12]

Even if you were reared by psychologically sound, secure parents, you no doubt learned to deny some of your own needs in order to please them or other people who were important to you. Such splitting from certain aspects of your fully integrated, natural self is shaped by the expectations of parents and significant others, and by your own intuition about what you need to do in order to either gain praise (looks or words of approval), avoid punishment (criticism or discipline), or escape negative states (the distress or anxiety of others). The result is explained by psychologist Marion Solomon:

> Aspects of the self deemed unacceptable, those filled with the child's needs, intense emotions, or thoughts, may have to be denied or left underdeveloped in exchange for being loved by the parents. While appearing mature at an early age, and presenting a strong outward appearance, such children hold in feelings of longing.[13]

Identifying Your Splits

To identify the drivers described earlier, you must pinpoint what you were taught to *do* in order to be accepted and loved. This usually comes from a combination of advice, warnings, and role modeling.

To identify your splits, on the other hand, you must pinpoint what you learned *not* to express in order to gain acceptance and love. This most often comes from subtle cues, recognized from intuition (which may or may not have been accurate).

In identifying the specific content of splits, it is helpful to recall your childhood notions of what sorts of thoughts, feelings, and needs were safe to express. Specifically, it is helpful to recall or imagine the reactions of parents and significant others to childlike expressions of a wide range of natural emotions. The following exercise is designed to help you pinpoint the influences that in this way might have shaped your psychological splits.

Splitting Origins Exercise[14]

Take a few minutes to relax your body and mind. Inhale deeply and hold your breath for a moment. Next, fully exhale as you see and hear the word "relax" slowly unfold. Let yourself enjoy a tranquil, peaceful moment as you become aware of the pull of gravity on your body. Relax each of your body parts and clear your mind.

In this state of relaxed concentration, recall your family home during the years of your youth. Think especially of a time when you were around seven years old. If you lived in more than one place during those years, simply choose one of those homes and focus on it. Remember how it looked: How many rooms did it have? What was the floor plan? What type of floor and wall coverings did it have? Also recall the smells of your house and the sounds that you most often noticed while living there. Next, recall the atmosphere of your childhood home. Was it a cozy, warm place or a cold, sterile environment?

In your mind's eye, imagine your family as it was at this stage of your childhood. Who was living in this home with you? Picture each person in your family as they were at that stage of your life.

Now imagine a typical evening in your family, after everyone had returned home from the day's activities. Notice where in the house the different people in your family are. Who is doing what? Hold on to these images.

Next, as that seven-year-old, imagine yourself outdoors, walking up your driveway toward your home. You enter the front door and are faced with the following scenarios. (One at a time, notice your reactions to each of the following scenes. Start each scene by backing up your fantasy and, once again, as a youngster, enter your childhood home and interact with your family in the ways described below. As you think of these scenarios, notice what is reacted to and how these reactions make you feel—about yourself and about the thoughts, feelings, or behaviors that you are expressing. Also notice how different family members react to you in each scene.)

Scene 1: You burst through the door, bustling with playful energy. Laughing and joking, you say hello to your family.

Notice who reacts to you and how that reaction affects you in the fantasy.

Scene 2: This time, you slowly open the door and enter your home, slouched and shuffling. Tears fill your eyes as you whimper to your family that you are sad. Something has happened between you and your best friend that has hurt your feelings.

Who reacts how?

Scene 3: You storm into the house, angrily slamming the door behind you. You are furious. A teacher treated you unfairly at school today, and you are angry enough to kill.

Who reacts how?

Scene 4: Again, you storm angrily into the house. This time, the target of your anger is a friend who double-crossed you on the playground.

Who reacts how?

Scene 5: You storm angrily into the house, slam the door, and—with outrage in your voice—remind your mother that she "forgot" to do something that she had promised she would.

Who reacts how?

Scene 6: You storm angrily into the house, slam the door, and—with outrage in your voice—remind your father that he "forgot" to do something that he had promised he would.

Who reacts how?

Scene 7: You enter the house whistling. Cheerfully, you greet everyone, and you spontaneously offer hugs and kisses.

Who reacts how?

Scene 8: You come into the house like a little adult. You greet everyone, efficiently put your things away, and get on with the business of doing your chores or homework.

Who reacts how?

Scene 9: You enter your home with an audible sigh of relief. "I'm so glad I'm home. I'm ready to watch television and just play!"

Who reacts how?

Scene 10: You slowly enter your home and gently shut the door. You don't feel well; you have a headache, a tummyache, and are "just feeling sick."

Who reacts how?

Scene 11: You come home beaming with pride. You gleefully announce, "I got a prize for being the best today!"

Who reacts how?

Scene 12: You enter your house, obviously bothered by something. "I'm really worried. I don't know what to do."

Who reacts how?

Scene 13: You enter your house, run up to your family (or to a given family member), and jumping up and down, blurt out: "I've got a secret! I've got a secret! Want me to tell you?"

Who reacts how?

Scene 14: You come home, relax a bit, and get into conversation with your family. In the conversation you respectfully question some firmly stated opinion or belief of your parents with a statement like "It seems to me that there might be another way of thinking about this. How about . . ."

Who reacts how?

Which expressions on your part led to reactions that were shaming, critical, cold, blaming, preaching, ignoring, chiding, tired, overwhelmed, anxious, afraid, sarcastic, or abusive? What kinds of thoughts, feelings, or actions on your part led to reactions that were warm, loving, playful, affirming, nurturing, encouraging, helpful, permissive, indicative of pride in you, or approving of you?

Our purpose in presenting this exercise is to help you begin to identify the emotional, cognitive, and behavioral substitutions that signal your version of psychological splitting. Which forms of thinking, feeling, and acting did you learn to emphasize? Which did you learn to minimize? What we learned to minimize in our past is what we tend to want permission to actualize in our present relationships.

When you find yourself struggling in your marriage, it is safe and useful to assume that your struggle is at least partially due to two factors: (1) your overuse of your most familiar ("good self") personality-based coping patterns, and (2) the frustrations and pains that have accumulated from downplaying your unexpressed (split off) traits.

We are creatures who gravitate toward the familiar. We feel comforted by familiar surroundings, cultures, smells, and tastes, and by familiar ways of thinking, acting, perceiving, and interacting. Most people organize their lives to create and maintain familiarity.

It therefore makes sense that we might have difficulty convincing ourselves that it is both wise and safe to try something new and different in the midst of the gut-level alarm we feel when we face stressful times in our intimate relationships. We are especially likely to shy away from openly expressing thoughts or feelings that reside in our underdeveloped selves, given the punishment we have received in the past for just such expression.

Remaining locked into self-defeating coping patterns can sabotage our efforts to renegotiate our relationship contracts, confuse us as we try to declare our differences from our loved ones, and even keep us from turning to our loved ones for help and support during times of crisis. Many of us, like Christine in the following case example, keep on trying the same coping strategies (even though they may not be working) simply because the alternatives are uniquely uncomfortable.

Christine learned early in life that Being Strong *and* Trying Hard *were essential in her quest to feel good about herself. These traits served her well throughout her medical training and residency in oncology and in her dealings with the sometimes sexist world of medical education and practice; also, in facing the shock that came when her husband, Alan, found out he had colon cancer at the age of fifty-one.*

Following her husband's diagnosis, Christine never shed a tear or showed any signs of distress. She simply went about her days, working hard to be a source of strength to her husband and children and a source of financial security to her family.

All went well until this strong woman began experiencing chest pains. For months she tried to ignore them, just as she had ignored her emotional pain. But when her discomfort grew to the point of interfering with her breathing, she was frightened into consulting a cardiologist.

Christine was diagnosed with mild hypertension and angina. Her physician warned that the stress of her life might be complicating her health. She was encouraged to begin expressing her feelings more openly and to ask for and accept support from her family and friends during this stressful period of life. However, her chest pains continued to plague her over the next six months, and her physician eventually referred her to our clinic for stress-management training.

Christine was uncomfortable with being referred to a "shrink." After all, she was accustomed to using her own willpower to work through her problems. But she was also a sensible woman, concerned about her health and courageous enough to examine her own coping struggles. She explained her reactions to her physician's advice this way:

"As I was driving home from my doctor's office after that first visit, I realized how scared and alone I had been feeling since my husband's diagnosis. I even cried a few tears. It was true that I felt all pent up with tension.

"I decided that I would start expressing my feelings more. I surely didn't want to die from a heart attack! My kids were going through enough with their father's cancer; they didn't need to have a sick mother to boot.

"So I went home and told Alan that I was scared and tired and that this whole ordeal was hard on me, too. I did what my doctor said to do, and it didn't work.

"I felt even worse when Alan started crying and blaming himself for being a burden on me. I also felt weak and stupid, sitting there crying on my sick husband's shoulder. So how was I supposed to get this 'support' that my doctor was telling me I needed? I was not going to lean on my kids, and I don't believe in talking about my personal life with my friends.

"After 'expressing myself' to my husband, I couldn't sleep for two nights, plus I still had chest pains! I decided to go back to keeping my mouth shut and bearing through the pain myself. At least this way only one of us is suffering. I can't stand it when I upset Alan or my children."

Is Change Really Possible?

We all face a fundamental problem here: Most people doubt that anyone can truly change their personality in any lasting way. They believe that internal psychological struggles, such as low self-esteem or irritability, may last a lifetime.

We won't argue this last point. Indeed, longitudinal studies of adults have shown that certain personality traits, such as extroversion or neuroticism, remain stable over periods of time ranging from six to forty-five years. Our early life experiences do often leave us thinking about ourselves and others in ways that seem indelibly recorded in our brains.

These overlearned perspectives can privately haunt us even once we have objectively changed. For example, reformed alcoholics often secretly feel fraudulent as sober people, although they may not have tasted alcohol in many years. A thin adult may feel like a "fat kid in disguise," even though he or she has not been overweight in many years. Outgoing, socially skillful people sometimes admit that they secretly are very shy, a self-description that is often based on an earlier life filled with painful experiences that came from their social awkwardness.

The power of old, internalized self-descriptions may last a lifetime. However, you *can* learn to cope differently when reacting to your internal struggles, just as you can learn new behaviors when coping with the stresses of your daily life. In other words, even if your personality is not changeable, your personality-based coping patterns *are* changeable.

Five Keys to Changing Personality-based Coping Patterns

The experiences of Christine in the preceding case study highlight five important facts about the hard work of psychological and relationship growth.

1. Changing old coping patterns often means changing old relationship patterns.
2. Such changes may not feel good at first. Healthy changes often stir feelings of awkwardness—both internally and in relationships. Making healthy changes may lead to fears that you are making things worse by stressing yourself and your loved ones with these new ways of behaving.
3. This initial anxiety and awkwardness does not mean that changing is a mistake; it simply signals that you are in new and unfamiliar territory, both as an individual and as a couple. The more you behave in this new, more healthy way, the more familiar and comfortable it will become.
4. You must remain open and communicative with each other as you change. Including loved ones in any exploration of a new way of living is crucial if you want to improve your relationship as you improve yourself.
5. A key factor in beating stress together is asking for support when attempting any sort of change. We especially need support from each other in attempting to change personality-based coping patterns.

Helping Each Other Cope

How do you identify what type of support to give and to ask for? Learn to recognize and respond to the hopes and needs that underlie each of the personality drivers.

The behaviors that come with each of the personality drivers usually mask underlying hopes and needs. If you learn to soothe each other's underlying hopes and needs, you will accomplish two important tasks in your relationship. First, by responding to the underlying need, rather than the expressed behavior, you are more likely to solve the problem rather than perpetuate or worsen it. Second, by soothing each other in these fundamental ways, you will become a unique source of intimate connection for each other; your relationship will become a safe haven in which each of you can risk change by incorporating appropriate expressions of these split-off aspects of yourselves into your life. The result will be a more flexible, safe, loving relationship.

Coping Patterns and Underlying Hopes

Identify the underlying needs and hopes that correspond with each of the personality drivers.

Driver	Underlying Hope
Being Strong	To be nurtured
Being Perfect	To feel good enough
Trying Hard	To feel deserving of rest and enjoyment
Pleasing Others	To feel understood and appreciated
Hurrying	To feel finished
Being Careful	To feel safe

Each of the coping drivers is accompanied by underlying hopes that are not obvious from the behaviors that typify the driver pattern. For example, the hope underlying *Being Strong* is the wish to be nurtured. But when we act strong, we convey the message that we do not need anything from anyone. Eventually, we end up stuck in a coping pitfall signaled by the stress symptoms outlined above.

For example, high-powered people driven by *Being Strong* end up feeling lonely and numb. Often a vicious cycle ensues which can last a lifetime and thwart growth in any relationship. As we drive ourselves harder and harder, we continue to misrepresent our underlying needs and therefore continue to experience the frustration of not getting these needs met. Soon we lose sight of the part we play in perpetuating our discomfort and misinterpret our driver-caused pain as an indication that something is wrong with the way we are being treated by our mates.

Again, an example, using the *Being Strong* driver: The more you act strong, the less you convey that you need nurturing. The less nurturing you get from others, the more lonely you feel. The more lonely you feel, the more numb you become. The more numb you feel, the stronger you act, the less support you elicit from others. Eventually, your most intimate relationship may begin to feel like the *cause* of your loneliness. You defend yourself against this disappointing relationship by developing further numbness, a defense that simply serves to thwart intimacy in your life. Your most important relationships can seem like the most wounding source of rejection of your most fundamental emotional needs.

When you notice yourself feeling or acting in ways that are suggested in the "stress symptoms" column of the chart on page 54, try asking for support that might soothe your corresponding underlying hope, as specified in the chart on page 62. For example, if you feel exhausted and joyless, it may be that you are stuck in a *Trying Hard* driver. You may be having difficulty giving yourself permission to take your fair share of rest and enjoyment. Asking for a supportive reminder from a trusted loved one that you do deserve rest and enjoyment will make it easier to do what is necessary to recoup your energies.

Similarly, if you notice a loved one acting in ways described in the "stress symptoms" column, you can react in a more nurturing way. For example, if your partner is obsessing, preoccupied with feelings of guilt and anxiety about a given problem (indicating that he or she is stuck in *Being Perfect*), you might offer encouragement that he or she is making good enough progress in dealing with the problem at hand. Or, if your partner is fearful and worrying without any specific focus to his or her concerns (indicating pain from *Being Careful*), you might offer the calming message that things will work out and a feeling of safety is forthcoming.

We are not encouraging you to assume responsibility for solving your partner's problems. We are simply encouraging you to act like a loving partner. Notice signs that your mate is struggling and try to be soothing where he or she hurts most.

Is Trying to Change How I Cope Really Worth It?

The answer to this question is a definite *yes!* When you are trapped in any single pattern of coping, you lose flexibility and power. In this state, you are not in charge of when and how you react. Anyone—even a perfect stranger—can push your buttons, turning on your overlearned style of reacting simply by frustrating you. Once you lock into reflexive use of a single coping pattern, you lose control of your own internal emotional or physical experience and of the effect you are having on other people.

Finally, it is important to underscore that no coping pattern is innately "bad" or "good." The important question is, what effect is your coping pattern having on your life? The answer depends on how the coping pattern is used. It is adaptive to have your most familiar tools in your arsenal of coping strategies. It is even more important to learn when *not* to use each of these tools.

The goal is to be more selective about how and when you use your different coping capabilities. Learning to do so will minimize destructive relationship "tricks," like displacement and projection, that can otherwise sabotage growth in your marriage.

References

1. Hendrie KH, Clair DK, Brittain HM, Fadul PE. A study of anxiety/depressive symptoms of medical students, house staff, and their spouses/partners. *J Nerv Ment Dis.* 1990;178:204-207.
2. Firth-Cozens J. Sources of stress in women junior house officers. *BMJ.* 1990;301:89-91.
3. Krakowski AJ. Stress and the practice of medicine: the myth and the reality. *J Psychosom Res.* 1982;26:91-98.
4. Sacks MH, Frosh WA, Kesselman M, Parker L. Psychiatric problems in third year medical students. *Am J Psychiatry.* 1980;137:822-825.
5. Sakinofsky I. Suicide in doctors and wives of doctors. *Can Fam Phys.* 1980;26:837-844.
6. Vaillant G, Sobawale NC, McArthur C. Some psychologic vulnerabilities of physicians. *N Engl J Med.* 1972;287:372-375.
7. Roy A. Suicide in doctors. *Psychiatr Clin North Am.* 1985;8:377-387.
8. Miles JE, Krell R, Lin T-Y. The doctor's wife: mental illness and marital pattern. *Int J Psychiatry Med.* 1975;64:481-487.
9. Gabbard GO, Menninger RW. *Medical Marriages.* Washington, DC: American Psychiatric Press, Inc; 1988.
10. Krakowski AJ. Stress and the practice of medicine, II: physicians compared with lawyers. *Psychother Psychosom.* 1984;42:143-151.
11. Olsen RD, Sande JR, Olsen GP. Maternal parenting stress in physicians' families. *Clin Pediatr.* 1991;30:586-590.
12. Miller A. *The Drama of the Gifted Child: The Search for the True Self.* New York, NY: Basic Books; 1981:34.
13. Solomon MF. *Narcissism and Intimacy: Love and Marriage in an Age of Confusion.* New York, NY: WW Norton; 1989:74.
14. Thanks to Vann Joinnes, Ph.D., Director of the Southeast Institute in Chapel Hill, North Carolina, for introducing us to this helpful exercise.

Chapter 4

Type A Behavior Pattern and Medical Marriage

> Staying *the course is not at all the same as* enjoying *the course.*
>
> —**Leon Eisenberg, M.D.,** Harvard Medical School

Two beliefs shape much of our work with medical couples: First, the stresses described in the preceding chapters lead most physicians and their spouses to develop some version of Type A behavior pattern (TYABP). Furthermore, TYABP is not only a *result* of, but also a frequent *cause* of the stresses in a medical marriage. The "hurry sickness" that is inherent in TYABP can exaggerate or magnify any of the coping drivers discussed in Chapter 3.

What Is TYABP?

Cardiologists Meyer Friedman and Ray Rosenman originated the concept of TYABP from their observations of their hard-driving heart patients.[1] Specifically, they noted that their patients often seemed stuck in a lifestyle of struggling: these patients aggressively struggled to achieve more and more in less and less time, and they justified their struggling with the worldview that the environment is a hostile or limiting place filled with incompetent people. Furthermore, they seemed convinced that other people were invested in opposing their progress—a perception that further justified their constant struggling.

This conviction that one must struggle through life seems to fuel the coping habits that broadly characterize the Type A syndrome, but there is no precise way to describe TYABP. The variations of this coping pattern are limitless. TYABP does not refer to a set personality *trait*. It is a *way of coping* that consists of many factors, at least some of which will emerge in *any* person who is placed in the wrong situation long enough. Some people develop certain aspects of TYABP and not others; some show TYABP in certain situations and not in others.[2]

A list of psychological and behavioral characteristics that have been earmarked by contemporary researchers as typifying TYABP follows. We hope that you will not use this list to label yourself or each other; our intention here is not to encourage any form of character assassination. Don't use the information to blame or shame. Rather, use it to empower yourself to take more nurturing control of yourself and of your relationships.

As you read through the list, take note of descriptions that apply to you and those that describe your partner. Also note the situations that are most likely to stir your Type A reactions. And remember: These are *general* characteristics of TYABP; the list is not exhaustive. Note what needs to be added or subtracted from the list to accurately describe *your* coping style.

Summary of Type A Response Styles*
The Type A[+] individual is driven by:
Conscientiousness and an inflexible sense of responsibility

Perfectionism

High levels of cynicism and hostility

The need to prove self-worth through performing well

Cravings for recognition and power

Competition and challenges

Driving need to work long, hard hours

The desire to be seen as a leader

A vague mistrust of the motives or competency of others

The Type A behaviors include:
Tense, energetic movements

Constant movement: difficulty being still. Fidgeting, tapping feet, drumming knuckles, or shaking leg or foot while attempting to sit still

Explosively emphasizing points during conversation with finger and hand motions

Frequent uses of profanity

Forceful expressions of opinions, often using such words as "stupid," "idiotic," and "ridiculous" in response to opinions differing from one's own

Flashing grimacelike smiles

A clipped speaking pattern, the result of constantly tensing jaw muscles

Irregular breathing pattern, often leading to expiratory sighs in the midst of conversations

Constantly rushing and fighting against time—also known as hurry sickness

Overly aggressive and competitive reactions even when the situation does not warrant such

Doing several things at once

The Type A's style and focus of thinking:

Tends to think on several levels at once

Anticipates what is coming next and reacts in advance (Examples: interrupts conversations with answers to unfinished questions or prepares for departure from car or airplane well before the vehicle stops)

Hypervigilant: scans surroundings, noticing what might go wrong or what is irritating at the moment

Constantly checks the time, noting time crunch, punctuality (own or others'), and efficiency (or lack thereof)

Preoccupation with all of the above results in poor observational abilities, especially of one's own behavior or of the impact of one's own behavior on others

Factors that affect interpersonal relationships for Type A's:

Self-focused: preoccupied with own stresses, anxieties, or tasks

Poor listener: interrupts, breaks rapport with distracted behavior, gives advice rather than empathy

Easily bored by another's conversation

Easily angered and has difficulty not showing it (glaring, curt comments, or honking the horn at others while driving)

Makes critical, blaming, or shaming comments when someone makes a mistake

Defensive in reacting to feedback, especially regarding obvious hostility

Shows overt bravado and confidence regarding own opinions, abilities, and power

Often frustrated when working with others

Very controlling: dictates, gives unsolicited advice

Visibly uncomfortable with physical intimacy or with verbal expressions of tender feelings

*Adapted with permission from: Sotile WM. *Heart Illness and Intimacy: How Caring Relationships Aid Recovery.* Baltimore, Md: Johns Hopkins University Press; 1992:166-167.

†Like most authors on this subject, we will use phrases such as "the Type A" in referring to a person who habitually evidences some variant of TYABP in coping with stress simply to facilitate reading. We again emphasize that TYABP does not represent a distinct personality "type." It is a style of *coping* with stress that comes in many flavors.

If you are stuck in a Type A style of coping—or in a relationship with someone with TYABP—you will relate to the words of Canadian psychologist Ethel Roskies. Perhaps more than anything, Roskies proposes, TYABP is an *inefficient use of powerful coping energy.* As she puts it:

> The Type A is more often at war than at peace, repeatedly mobilizing his or her resources to confront perceived threats and challenges. A game of tennis, a difference of opinion with a colleague at work, and a too-slow elevator all produce a stress reaction in the hypersensitive Type A. . . . Even a nonstressful environment [will] be perceived and reacted to as challenging by the hyperreactive Type A. There are no safe environments for the person who engages in mortal combat even during a "friendly" game of tennis![3]

Does This Stuff Really Apply to Medical Marriages?

We believe that unless it is controlled, TYABP will magnify any of the personality-based driver patterns described in Chapter 3. For example:

- The stress-hardy individual whose *Being Strong* personality typically serves him or her well can go numb in an ever-escalating flurry of Type A reactivity.
- As TYABP gets more intense, orderly people are at risk of becoming compulsively driven toward *Being Perfect* behavior.
- The relentless drive to achieve that comes with TYABP can push *Trying Hard* tendencies into workaholism.
- The Type A-driven need for approval from others can lead the typically *Pleasing Others* person to live as though life is a quest to be all things to all people.
- The hurry sickness inherent in TYABP can propel a person already scripted to *Hurrying* into a lifestyle of free-floating anxiety and irritability.
- The typically cautious person can become quasi-paranoid as his or her Type A-driven anxieties amplify his or her *Being Careful* personality or her scripting.

Perhaps due to the various ways that one can "catch" TYABP, we have counseled just as many nonprofessional Type A homemakers as Type A workaholic physicians.

Where Does TYABP Come From?

It is easy to hypothesize but difficult to prove any single answer to this question. Each of the following perspectives on the origins of TYABP has merit.

Answer 1: The Environment Made Me Do It. Most people will develop one flavor or another of Type A coping style if placed in the "wrong" environment for long enough. In fact, research has shown that upwards of 70 percent of individuals who live in urban populations (and only a slightly smaller percentage of inhabitants of rural populations) develop at least one pronounced sign of TYABP.[4] Any workplace, home, or society that is filled with demands to compete, rush, and adapt to security-threatening levels of stress and strain can foster TYABP.

Certainly, medical training and medical workplaces overflow with Type A-promoting factors. Working as a physician virtually *guarantees* a lifestyle filled with situations or people that compel you to rush, to be constantly aware of time passing, to try to control outcomes, to do and think more than one thing at once, to compete, and so forth. The result?

It is very difficult to become a physician without also becoming Type A.

Indeed, research has documented that simply going through medical school promotes TYABP, and that physicians are exposed to more Type A-promoting experiences (like time pressures and threats to their control) than are such other medical professionals as dentists.

Cross-cultural research has also shown that, compared to the general population, physicians have elevated scores on measures of TYABP.[5,6] Female physicians seem to be at particular risk of developing TYABP. While Type A scores of the general public tend to be lower in women than in men, female physicians have more pronounced TYABP than male physicians and significantly elevated TYABP scores in comparison to women in the general public. For both sexes, TYABP is more prevalent in surgeons, pediatricians, and obstetricians than in psychiatrists. Whether the presence of TYABP predisposes some individuals to choose certain areas of specialization or the demands of working in certain medical specialties promote TYABP is not clear.

If you spend time in a relationship with a Type A, your own behavior will shift in Type A directions. This is because relationship "teams" organize around the most consistent themes in the relationship.

We work with many high-powered people who endure the following sequence: First, their early-learned coping patterns predispose them to become superachievers. Accordingly, they gravitate toward excessively demanding educational or training environments that foster TYABP.

Once educated and credentialed, they continue to work in environments that promote TYABP. In addition, their *own* TYABP gradually shapes the tones and patterns of other arenas (such as their family and friendship circles), even when these arenas are *not* innately driven by Type A demands.

Both partners in many contemporary medical marriages undergo this same process at once. The result? A relationship that cascades into ever-increasing levels of TYABP due to the relentless activity that fills their life together—work, home, relationship, and social environments.

Answer 2: My Mama and Daddy Made Me Do It. It has been proposed that TYABP develops out of insecurities that come from early life experiences that teach one to focus on performance in order to earn a momentary sense of well-being, and that it is fueled by a never-ending need to prove oneself.[7] This theory is fueled by observations of the interactions between parents and children who show signs of TYABP as early as age three. Parents of Type A children tend to criticize more than praise their children's performance, give approval unpredictably or only when the children perform exceptionally, model TYABP themselves, project their own insecurities onto their children, and drive the children with messages to Be Strong, Be Perfect, Try Harder, and Hurry Up. Such influences can result in an uncertain sense of self-worth that is both masked and, at least momentarily, soothed by TYABP.

Whether or not physicians tend to come from families that promoted TYABP is a question that remains to be answered by future researchers. The sparse research that has been published regarding the childhood experiences of physicians gives at best only a sketchy picture of this topic. For example, the aforementioned landmark study by George Vaillant reported that only one third of physicians (compared to one half of controls) were rated as having had "good" childhoods.

Answer 3: My Genes Made Me Do It. Many people seem to experience a form of physical stress response that makes it difficult for them *not* to react with TYABP. A typical stress reaction begins when the autonomic nervous system triggers a sympathetic response of fight or flight upon encountering stress. This is the body's way of being "in sympathy" with a person when he or she faces a challenge; it prepares a person either to fight or flee. Once the challenge passes, the stress response is turned off by the calming influence of the parasympathetic branch of the autonomic nervous system, and the stress event is over.

Some Type A's experience problems on both ends of this typical stress response. When faced with stress—*especially stress that strips them of control or that interpersonally challenges them*—some Type A's experience exaggerated fight-or-flight responses. Their bodies pump out larger doses of adrenaline and other hormones than are needed to meet the challenge. Worse yet, some of these same people get very little physiological help in calming down once they are in full-fledged fight or flight. Their parasympathetic calming reaction is impaired. Their body readily turns on, but does not easily turn off, the stress response.[8]

Answer 4: You Made Me Do It. Type A's tend to accumulate frustrating experiences. People disturb them; they annoy people.

In the words of one of our patients:

Let me explain. Type A stands for Aggravated. *What with? Type B, B, B, B! As in: 'Move your Big slow Behind out of my way so I can get about my Business and lower my Blood pressure!'*

- Type A's tend to selectively perceive others as challenging them.
- Despite their often gruff and insensitive behavior, Type A's tend to be hypersensitive to criticism.
- Type A's react competitively in small groups, especially when dealing with other people who show TYABP.

- If open conflict with another person occurs, the Type A tends to show an initial flurry of reactivity as he or she tries to regain control of the relationship process. This is especially likely if the conflict crept up unexpectedly and if the reason for the conflict seems vague to the Type A. Type A's do not like unpredicted loss of control of relationships or ambiguous stress. They like to know whom to blame when they're miserable!
- If control is *not* regained by their initial flurry of TYABP, they shut down by withdrawing from further interactions.

In these ways, Type A's may perpetuate self-fulfilling prophecies: they assume that getting along with others is difficult; then they act and react in ways that prove this point, vacillating between overresponding and underresponding when interacting with others. These ways of reacting can simultaneously generate interpersonal conflict *and* impede conflict resolution.[9]

The ways that underlying beliefs shape TYABP are summarized in the following table, taken from *Heart Illness and Intimacy: How Caring Relationships Aid Recovery.*

Type A Beliefs and Behaviors

Believing that	The Type A acts
"I must constantly prove myself"	As if life is an endless struggle
"My sense of well-being is always in jeopardy"	Hostile
"Others can take away my self-worth"	Competitive and jealous and critical of self and other.
"I am not as talented as others"	As if he or she must always try harder than others
"Good may not prevail in the world"	Suspicious of the intentions of others
"All resources are scarce"	Urgently competitive

The Type A Triad

Such beliefs set the stage for what researcher Virginia Price has called the Type A triad.[7] This refers to the Type A's tendency to bounce back and forth among three states that shape thoughts, behaviors, and physiological responses: the *superperson* state, the *depressed* state, and the *angry* state.

The Superperson State

In the *superperson* state, the Type A is driven to prove to an imaginary or real audience that he or she is worthy of high regard and is capable of managing tremendous levels of stress and responsibility. The Type A responds to challenges with energy, vision, ambition, urgency, and commitment. During bursts of activity that fill the superperson state, the

Type A focuses only on the tasks at hand. The environment and the people in it may be ignored or responded to with irritation if they thwart progress. It is during the superperson state that Type A's often look and act like workaholics. They ignore signs of increasing physical or mental fatigue.

Any human being living this way will eventually begin to experience burnout, one sign of which is increased sensitivity to any negative life event. Accordingly, living in the superperson state sets Type A's up to avalanche into the second stage of the Type A triad—the depressed state.

The Depressed State

The Type A's *depressed* state is usually triggered abruptly by some setback: a spouse's criticism, a missed deadline, failure to reach a goal, or an illness. Such events confront us with our inability to control life totally. This is especially painful for any Type A. When forced to acknowledge his or her lack of control, the Type A experiences a variant of depression that has been termed "vital exhaustion"—a state characterized by overwhelming self-blame and discouragement, fear that life's obstacles will not be overcome, paralyzing levels of distress, and atypical passivity in responding to the challenges at hand.

This depressed state creates a dilemma for Type A's. Because they tend to interpret feelings of sadness and vulnerability as signs of weakness, Type A's also blame and shame themselves when they really need soothing that can only come from self-nurturing or from accepting others' support. Their excessively high standards and tendency to selectively perceive negative feedback propel them into a momentary state of helplessness and depression.

Making themselves feel worse by their own self-criticism and not knowing how to cope with these feelings, Type A's may resort to pseudo-solutions for their pain. They may momentarily distract themselves by switching back to the superperson state. Or, more often, they embrace the following motto: "When things go wrong, find out whom to blame and blame that sucker!" Accordingly, the next stage of the Type A triad involves switching into the angry state.

The Angry State

Given that Type A's have difficulty trusting in their own or others' inherent goodness, it is easy to see how they might assume that others think badly of them, especially when they are less than perfect. Type A's tend to project their own negative self-judgments onto others. When they feel depleted, insecure, or depressed, they assume that others (e.g., spouses, bosses, or coworkers) are criticizing them. They then act on the anger that comes from this assumption. Being angry brings temporary relief from feelings of vulnerability and can become a habitual substitution. If any self-doubt or vulnerability surfaces, anger is triggered. Interestingly, during this angry state, Type A's almost always report feeling victimized and therefore justified in their anger. The anger does not feel good; but at least it feels better than fear, vulnerability, or depression.

The Relationship Between TYABP and High-Poweredness

We believe that most high-powered people are Type A in one way or another. However, not all Type A's are high-powered.

In his groundbreaking work, psychologist Warren Farrell notes that power is related to the ability to clarify one's expectations and then meet them in five areas:

- Such external rewards as income, status, and possessions
- Such internal rewards and resources as inner peace
- Interpersonal contact
- Physical health, attractiveness, and intelligence
- Sexual fulfillment[10]

Many extreme Type A reactors do not succeed in any of these areas. They are like high-powered machines that are out of control. Their random bursts of overcharge render them ineffectual as they waste their energy reacting to every stress as though life itself were at stake. They work hard but do not accomplish their goals. The more they flounder rather than accomplish, the more their frustrations boost their TYABP.

Other Type A's are successful by objective standards, but they constantly *perceive themselves* to be failing due to their ever-increasing expectations. No matter how much they achieve, receive, or do, their accomplishments always pale in comparison to their expectations.

This process can take many forms. A few examples follow.

Jean, wife of an internist: *"My husband is constantly complaining that we do not have sex often enough. With three kids to raise, his career, and my exhaustion, what does he expect? The answer is 'more!' I guess that's just the way he is. That's okay. But here's the problem: Even when we do have a lot of sex, he always wants more. If we go away for a weekend and have sex repeatedly, he always approaches me again until I finally say no. It's like he isn't comfortable unless the scales stay tipped in the direction of his sexual expectations not being met."*

Mia, wife of a cardiologist: *"First he just wanted to make enough money to be able to afford a comfortable lifestyle. We did that. Then he felt urgent about making more money so we could 'get ahead of the wave' of upcoming expenses. We did that. Now he's obsessed with making even more money than he does—it doesn't really matter why. The point is that he's stuck in the quest to 'make more' no matter how much we've got."*

Rosana, an anesthesiologist: *"I made the decision not to have chil-dren until I finished my residency and got established in academic medi-cine. Well, I did both of those things. I just got tenured, and now I have a baby. But I am forty-three years old. I won't have another child. My heart breaks every time I see my sister—thirty-seven years old, mother of three growing kids, happy as a lark. I have to come to grips with this."*

People stuck in this trap never feel satisfied. They spend half their lives playing the "wait until" game and the other half lamenting what they do not have.

Does this mean that we are all doomed to unhappiness? Certainly not. The world of medical marriages is filled with healthy Type A's. We have worked with hundreds of happily married physicians and thousands of other thriving, vital people. A large body of research supports our clinical impressions that healthy Type A's are among the most happy, most con-tented, dynamic, and successful people. In general, studies have shown that TYABP does not necessarily correlate with subjectively rated signs of stress or with objectively measured degrees of neuroticism or other forms of psychopathology.[11] On the contrary, for some people, TYABP correlates with such personality traits as extroversion, self-confidence, and a height-ened sense of mastery and vigor in coping with stress. Type A behavior has also been associated with positive life experiences, such as success in school, career distinction, and high occupational status.

However, these "benefits" of TYABP do not apply to everyone.

It has been documented that females who show high levels of TYABP also report more emotional distress and frustration, poorer physical health, poorer marital adjustment, less self-esteem, and more general unhappiness than non-Type A women.[4,12] Women who identify with a more traditionally feminine role and lifestyle seem especially to suffer negative effects of their own TYABP. On the other hand, women who are characterized as highly Type A and who also show elevated levels of mas-culinity (as measured by standardized sex-role inventories) report greater self-esteem and less depression than their counterparts who are both Type A and more feminine.[13]

These facts may in part account for observed differences in the reac-tions of male versus female physicians to the stresses of medical practice. It seems that male physicians are more likely to be stressed by experi-ences that call into question their authority and status, such as noncom-pliant patients and claims of malpractice, and that they are likely to mani-fest symptoms of anxiety rather than depression. Women physicians, on the other hand, are more likely to report stress from their combined roles of career and family and are significantly more likely than their male col-leagues to report symptoms of depression.[14,15]

The relatively high distress levels of Type A women who identify with the feminine role may be due to societal prohibitions against females showing their own high-powered capabilities. It also may be that such Type A women are more honest and accurate than either their male counterparts or their more "macho" female counterparts in identifying the subjective stresses that come with the lifestyles that most Type A's construct.

In either case, the research with female Type A's indirectly makes an important point: In assessing TYABP, researchers tend to focus on *individual* issues, such as career success, satisfaction with one's station in life, and *individual* measures of psychological health. The point that is being missed in such research is that the most prevalent consequences of TYABP involve *relationship*, not individualistic, factors. The people who are most bothered by TYABP are the very people who tend to be our society's torch carriers when it comes to relationship intimacy—women who embrace a feminine point of view. Such women are likely to be adept at the *sine qua non* of feminine psychological development: attending to the needs of other people. Accordingly, the documented distress of a woman who is both Type A and feminine in psychological orientation points to an important fact about TYABP: If unchecked, it disrupts relationship harmony—the cornerstone of beating stress together.

In our experience, both males and females who have a healthy awareness of their more "feminine" personality traits tend to be distressed by TYABP—either their own, or their spouses'.

What makes the difference between those medical couples who thrive and those who struggle through life? The key lies in the ways TYABP is managed, on both individual and relationship levels.

Eight Rules for Managing TYABP and Medical Marriage

Unchecked, TYABP strains relationships, and stress in relationships fuels TYABP. A key to thriving as a medical couple is to integrate your Type A coping patterns into a lifestyle and relationship style that allow for a sense of balance and wholeness. You must help each other become healthy Type A's. In our experience, healthy, high-powered Type A's follow eight rules.

Rule 1

Be honest about your own TYABP. Where and how are you most Type A in your coping style? Research has shown that while Type A's tend to evaluate their degree of TYABP in work settings honestly and accurately, they are notorious for underestimating the effects of their TYABP on family relationships. Don't underestimate the extent to which your spouse or children are negatively affected by your TYABP.

Start by listening to yourself as you deal with your loved ones. Ask for feedback regarding your way of relating to them. You might even tape record an evening's conversation with your family, and then listen to the tape. Become aware of *how* your Type A reactions affect your relationships. Be particularly cautious about the following pitfalls:

- If you are constantly *in a hurry*, your connection with loved ones will be impaired.
- If you are constantly *doing more than one thing at once*, others will feel that you never fully attend to them.
- If you are *impatient*, others will feel anxious when around you.
- If you are *perfectionistic*, your criticism will alienate others.
- If you repeatedly show *irritation and hostility*, others will feel wounded, not nurtured, by you.
- If you are *controlling* in your interactions, others will stop revealing themselves to you, fearing another unwanted lecture.
- If you are excessively *competitive*, others will avoid spending time with you for fear of being put down.
- If you are frequently *exhausted* from your superperson quests, you will drain the vibrancy out of your family relationships.

Rule 2

Remember: Insecurity and anxiety, not haughtiness, power, or inflated self-worth, fuel TYABP. As you attempt to change these reactions, be nurturing to each other, not blaming or shaming.

Rule 3

Respect your Type A physiology. If you are Type A in your coping style, you cannot afford to fuel your already overly reactive central nervous system by ingesting excessive amounts of stimulants, such as caffeine, nicotine, and simple sugars. Avoid the trap that ensnares many Type A's: alternating use of stimulants to stoke their energies with some form of sedation in order to calm down. Excessive consumption of alcohol or food is a frequently used sedative in this syndrome.

A better—even essential—choice for any Type A is to engage in regular aerobic exercise, which relieves muscular tensions, provides distraction from worries, and triggers endorphins that aid relaxation and promote a sense of well-being. Research with Type A's has shown that regular exercise improves the ability to manage the fight-or-flight syndrome.[16]

A second way to respect your Type A physiology is to accept the need to relax. Research has repeatedly shown that Type A's mislabel or ignore their physical sensations.[8] For this reason, many Type A's claim to feel relaxed when objective measurements of body tension (such as muscular tightness and heart rate) indicate considerable stress.

Only when you learn to experience true physiological relaxation will you have a reference point from which to check yourself throughout the day for signs of growing tension. Learning and practicing a relaxation procedure is an essential step in understanding how and when your TYABP interferes with, rather than enhances, your coping.

Rule 4

Practice becoming a better environmental engineer. Once you honestly evaluate yourself, you will notice how often you unnecessarily use all of your Type A power in reacting to stress. Experiment with responding in non-Type A ways. Force yourself to drive slowly while listening to a relaxation tape or soft music. When there is no reason to rush, stand in the longest line at a checkout counter and spend the time in the line thinking pleasant thoughts about your past, present, or future. Limit the number of things you do at once: turn off the radio or television, put away reading material, and simply sit and talk with a loved one for a while. Practice doing nothing for fifteen-minute stints of time in order to get more familiar with slowing your pace.

By developing a more relaxed, accepting, in-control way of reacting, you will gain important coping leverage—the power to choose *how* and *when* you will react.

Rule 5

Manage hurry sickness. In *Beat Stress Together*, we made the point that you can neither manage TYABP nor maintain caring connection with others unless you resist the pull into chronic urgency that comes with a busy life. The realistic key here is to slow down in spurts. Family researcher Peter Fraenkel recommends that you pause briefly—even 20 seconds will do—between tasks, rather than overlapping and multitasking throughout the day.[17] Develop the habit of doing one thing at once when possible. Break up your busy day with brief moments of self-care or connection with loved ones. Family therapists David Waters and J. Terry Saunders made the point that phone calls, faxes, pagers, and express mail compress our lives and disconnect us from others.[18] Why not program a "call home and tell them you love them" message on your beeper or daily scheduler? These little changes can break up what otherwise will be escalating stress and withering connection with others as you go through your busy week.

Rule 6

Get out of your head and into your senses. If Type A's allow themselves to react "naturally," they almost always drift into thinking in ways that generate Type A reactivity. One way to counter this tendency is to fill your head with sensory awareness. Using all five of your senses as you notice your surroundings can be an interesting way to change your experience. Rather than driving to work in your typical tunnel of thinking, become aware of what is happening *right now*. What does the scenery look like? What do you hear and smell? How does your car's seat feel? Which parts of your body are more relaxed than other parts? Practice similar sensory awareness in brief spurts throughout the day as a way of slowing down and experiencing—rather than speeding through-your life. Apply these same sensory—awareness strategies during brief conversations, day-to-day routines, even during sex.

Rule 7

Practice empathy and compassion whenever you feel hostile. Many experts in TYABP believe that learning to be more compassionate is the key to curbing the most toxic element of TYABP—hostility.[19] Key here is controlling your thinking and your behavior, even if you cannot control your anger. First, notice what kinds of thoughts are fueling your anger. Most often these will have to do with perceiving someone as purposely frustrating you or convincing yourself that another will harm you if you are not careful. Even something as impersonal as another driver making a mistaken turn can be taken as a personal assault when you are lost in the blur of Type A reactivity.

When annoyed, most Type A's find it helpful to ponder questions that fuel compassion rather than anger. You might ask yourself: "I wonder what that person worries about?" "I wonder what kind of day that person has had?" "I wonder what frightens that person and makes him feel insecure?" "I wonder if anyone has been kind or courteous to that person today?"

It might also be helpful to remember certain phrases when you notice your anger rising. Remind yourself of the following: "Everyone just does the best that he or she can," or "No one has set out to annoy me; accidents and mistakes just sometimes happen," or "This won't affect the course of my life."

Perhaps most important in managing the effect that TYABP has on your family is to control your *behavior* regardless of what you think or feel. Don't fall prey to the most convenient rationalization for staying stuck in maladaptive ways of behaving in intimate relationships: "If it doesn't feel natural, then it isn't authentic and shouldn't be done." If you truly followed this bit of bad advice, you would never change anything. Remember: healthy change does not feel natural.

One of the guidelines in our *BEST* model for stress resilience is that you must remember that the change process is a process. Attitudinal (or conceptual) clarification regarding what you want to change and what you commit to changing comes first. Next comes behavioral practice, and only after many experiences of such practice will you feel emotionally comfortable with the decided-upon change. Remember, the change process goes as follows:

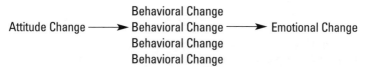

Put another way, we recommend that you not wait for it to feel different; make it different by *behaving* differently. Here we advise our clients to make healthy use of pretending. It's okay that you don't feel patient waiting for your wife to get dressed, just pretend that you are patient. It's all right that you don't feel tolerant when one of your loved ones makes an honest mistake; just pretend that you are nurturing rather than critical. It's okay that giving physical affection feels awkward; just pretend that you love doing it and do it a lot. If you pretend often enough, these "pretend" behaviors become a more natural and automatic way of reacting.

Rule 8

Find the courage to create non-Type A territory: relationships, situations, and processes that do *not* fuel your Type A reactivity. Remember that TYABP is largely a coping response to certain kinds of stimuli. For this reason, if you expose yourself to non-Type A stimuli, it will be easier to control your TYABP. Where possible, associate with people who soothe you, not with those who stir your competitive edge. Fill as much of your time as you can with activities that comfortably stimulate you, not with those that fuel your aggressive and hostile reactions. Learn to anticipate which situations and people are likely to push your TYABP buttons and, when possible, avoid them.

References

1. Friedman M, Rosenman RH. Type A behavior pattern: its association with coronary heart disease. *Ann Clin Res.* 1971;3:300-312.
2. Haynes SG, Matthews KA. Review and methodologic critique of recent studies on Type A behavior and cardiovascular disease. *Ann Behav Med.* 1988;10:47-59.
3. Roskies E. Type A intervention: where do we go from here? In: Strube MJ, ed. Type A Behavior. *J Soc Behav Pers.* 1990;5(special issue):419-438.

4. Thorensen CE, Low KG. Women and the Type A behavior pattern: review and commentary. In: Strube MJ, ed. Type A Behavior. *J Soc Behav Pers*. 1990;5(special issue):117-133.
5. Sterdoff B, Smith DF. Normal values for Type A behaviour patterns in Danish men and women and in potential high-risk groups. *Scand J Psychol*. 1990;31:49-54.
6. Smith DF, Sterdoff B. Female physicians outscore male physicians and the general public on type A scales in Denmark. *Behav Med*. 1991-92(Winter);17:184-189 .
7. Price V. *Type A Behavior Pattern: A Model for Research and Practice*. New York, NY: Academic Press; 1982.
8. Williams RB. *The Trusting Heart: Great News About Type A Behavior*. New York, NY: Time Books; 1989.
9. Sotile WM, Sotile MO. The angry physician, part 1: the temper-tantruming physician. *Phys Exec*. 1996;22:30-35.
10. Farrell W. *Why Men Are the Way They Are*. New York, NY: Berkley Books; 1986.
11. Rosenman RH. Type A behavior pattern: personal overview. In: Strube MJ, ed. Type A Behavior. *J Soc Behav Pers*. 1990;5(special issue):1-24.
12. Houston BK, Kelly KE. Type A behavior in housewives: relation to work, marital adjustment, stress, tension, health, fear-of-failure and self-esteem. *J Psychosom Res*. 1987;31:55-61.
13. DeGregorio E, Carver C. Type A behavior pattern, sex role orientation, and psychological adjustment. *J Pers Soc Psychol*. 1980;39:286-293.
14. Gross EB. Gender differences in physician stress. *JAMA*. 1992;47:107-114.
15. Firth-Cozens J. Sources of stress in women junior house officers. *BMJ*. 1990;301:89-91.
16. Blumenthal JA, Emery CF, Walsh MA, et al. Exercise training in healthy Type A middle-aged men: effects on behavioral cardiovascular responses. *Psychosom Med*. 1988;50:418-433.
17. Fraenkel P. The rhythms of couplehood: using time as a resource for change. *Fam Ther Networker*. 1996;200:65-77.
18. Waters D, Saunders T. I gave at the office. *Fam Ther Networker*. 1996;20:44-51.
19. Williams R, Williams V. *Anger Kills: Seventeen Strategies for Controlling the Hostility That Can Harm Your Health*. New York, NY: Time Books; 1993.

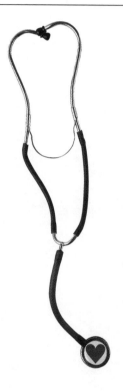

Part 2

The Basics of Love and Romance: Now and Forever

Chapter 5

How Do Relationships Grow?

We do not see things as they are. We see them as we are.
—Talmud

It all begins with so much innocence and good intention. As we chart our course in the world, we search for our One True Love. On this journey, most of us endure our fair share of false starts, which are usually more than innocent day trips: they hurt and frighten us, magnifying the drama that began as soon as we first realized the world into which we were born does not always respond perfectly to every need and desire. We eventually develop a quiet refrain that organizes much of our psychological and behavioral energy: "Will I be loved in a way that satisfies my needs and soothes my fears?"

If you are lucky, you find what appears to be your version of one true love—or at least a love that holds the promise and potential of becoming more true as your life together unfolds.

At the outset, your relationship promises to be your island of refuge amid the stresses of your collective lifestyle. Inevitably, this same relationship (and its many ramifications, including children, mortgages, businesses, careers, in-laws, and friendship networks, to name a few) seems to become the major *source of*, rather than the *solution to*, your respective stresses.

The way you manage yourself during critical passages determines whether your marriage endures as your most profound source of strength and support or becomes the most annoying source of stress.

Why Is This Happening to Us, of All People?

Seemingly endless variations of drama bring medical couples into our offices: concerns over children, stress from life changes, jealousies concerning a third party, fear about dwindling intimacy, frustrations about differences in sex drive or sexual likes and dislikes, efforts to gain support in making some seemingly healthy change in lifestyle, and more.

Most medical couples we meet believe their struggles are due to relatively small differences that should be easily negotiated. They come to counseling for help in problem solving, not out of a need for "serious headshrinking." As one of our favorite physician-clients once informed us:

Let's get something straight from the beginning. You are the third therapy type my wife has dragged me to during the past year, all because she thinks that the fact I am sick of being in private practice and want to go to work for an HMO indicates I have a screw loose. Now, what I want you to know right off the bat is what the last therapist 'discovered': When I was about 10 years old, I once walked into my parents' bedroom as my mother was getting dressed, and I saw her wearing nothing but her underwear. Let's get this straight: I don't think that my wanting to change careers has anything whatsoever to do with seeing my mama in her drawers. And if you *think it does, I'm leaving.*

Not all marriage problems have to do with childhood experiences that left deep psychological conflicts. Resolving relationship dilemmas does not require "serious headshrinking" for every couple.

But every medical marriage goes through complex developmental stages, and, minimally, every couple must deal with their fundamental differences and relative limitations to remain with their one true love. Many contemporary medical couples are vulnerable to a potentially fatal risk to relationship growth: they expect to be the exception to the rules that apply to all relationships.

In many ways, this makes sense. As high-powered people, partners in a medical marriage learn to expect more and produce more than others. They prove themselves to be exceptions to many rules. In order to learn to endure stress, some develop a self-centered urgency about circumventing anything that slows progress. Unfortunately, this sense of urgency usually compels them to avoid negotiating the developmental hurdles that must be overcome for any relationship to grow. As a dual-physician couple in marriage therapy expressed it: "We have proven to be the exceptions to many things. Why can't we just skip this mess about struggling to 'grow up' in our marriage and get on about the business of our life together?"

This brings us to a difficult but necessary concept, one that humbles even the most exceptional and high-powered couples: The day you join with another, you create a third party—your relationship system. This system takes on a life of its own. It operates largely according to universal rules that apply regardless of the makeup of the two of you. Accepting this concept is the beginning of growth for most medical couples, despite the current stage of the relationship.

Medical marriages are like houseplants: different versions of the species are inherently more beautiful, more hardy, and require more or less maintenance in order to survive and grow. But regardless of their innate differences, all plants share certain common characteristics. They need some degree of sunlight, water, and food in order to survive. Similarly, every relationship needs certain things to grow.

How Does a Medical Marriage Grow?

The teamwork of a long-term, intimate relationship is fascinating. Perhaps nowhere in life is the fact that we are creatures of habit more obvious than in our relationship patterns. We not only become locked into habitual ways of interacting with each other; we even grow accustomed to *perceiving* each other in certain ways. These perceptions resist change even when overwhelming data suggest that a fresh perspective would lead to a more accurate understanding of the other person and the relationship.

These perceptions and behavioral patterns constitute the relationship "contract" that organizes who you will be for each other and how you will live together as a couple. Several universal truths about relationship contracts are worth noting:

- Your original relationship contract serves a very useful purpose. It helps you to organize your behaviors and perceptions of each other in ways that allow you to join together to create a team that works.
- The original contract always relies on selective perception, wishful thinking, and well-intended but unrealistic hopefulness about who you will be in each other's life.
- The quality of your relationship depends on your ability to "renegotiate," periodically, the contract that organizes your perceptions, behaviors, attitudes, and emotional reactions to each other.

The Beginnings. Most romances begin in a blissful state of hero worship, narcissistic excitement, and intoxicating hope. We trust that this relationship will soothe each other's past emotional hurts and help to offset respective developmental hurdles. In this one true love, we believe we have finally found a partner who will make our dreams come true: each person's natural gifts will help the other overcome his or her own insecurities and become a more integrated person.

Nothing feels quite so wonderful and overwhelming as this first stage of love. Even our brain chemicals help to sweep us into ecstasy during infatuation. When we are first smitten by love, a flood of amphetamine-like substances (specifically, dopamine, norepinephrine, and phenylethylamine, or PEA) activate, stimulate, and motivate us. This same neurochemical bath sets into motion an interesting syndrome: pain receptors are blunted, needs for food and sleep seem to disappear, and mood and energy levels soar. When infatuated, we are motivated to do one thing above all else: win the love of *that person who is stirring all of this internal action!* It's as though this initial rush of neurochemicals renders us temporarily brain damaged. And in this state we make one of the most important decisions of our life: we choose a spouse.

One Whole Person. Given how intoxicating infatuation is, it is not surprising that at the outset of a new romance, we all see what we need to see and be what we need to be in order to create harmony. We view our new partner as our hope for being perfectly loved and see ourselves as a much-needed counterpart to our new partner. Each partner believes himself or herself to be a more complete and happy person.

In one way or another, most contemporary authorities on mate selection state that the one-true-love phenomenon is based on narcissistic processes that revolve around the psychological splitting phenomenon described in Chapter 3. Basically, these theories state, we choose a partner who "helps" us make contact with the disowned or underdeveloped parts of ourselves. In his eloquent book *The Fragile Bond*, family therapist Augustus Napier points out that it is the "unacknowledged part of ourselves which we recognize in our mate."[1(p225)]

Author Harville Hendrix, in his wonderful book *Keeping the Love You Find: A Guide for Singles*, notes that our one true love matches our stored images of the collective characteristics of caretakers and significant lovers from our past. Such a person stirs a primitive sense of familiarity in us. In the presence of this one true love, we automatically recall both the positive feelings and frustrated longings that resulted from these collective relationships.[2]

We tend to fall in love with someone who possesses traits that we have disowned, that we were taught were dangerous to the integrity of our expressed self. As Hendrix puts it:

> What you love in your partner is what you buried in yourself in order to survive. . . . What we unconsciously want is to get what we didn't get in childhood from someone who is like the people who didn't give us what we needed in the first place.[2(p165)]

The Contract That Binds. During the initial stage of romance, our thoughts, observations, fantasies, and conversations add clauses to a "contract" that organizes the relationship on both a behavioral and an emotional level. Much of the "negotiation" of the initial relationship contract is done consciously. For example, many of your early days together were no doubt spent discussing your likes, dislikes, past experiences, family dramas, emotional hurts and victories, dreams, future plans, and so forth. At that time, such discussions shaped images of what type of partner each of you wanted and needed, given who you were and what your life experiences had been up to that point.

In a state of infatuation, we all agree to be what our partner needs, even if doing so means leaving some parts of ourselves out of the relationship. The case of Beverly and Jim Warren demonstrates how this occurs.

The Warrens

We first met Beverly and Jim Warren when Jim was in his third year of a demanding residency in orthopedic surgery. We began our counseling of this couple by asking them to put words to their attraction to each other.

Jim was drawn to Beverly's combination of spunk, savvy, and nurturing caretaker style. Beverly began overachieving in grade school. She accomplished one "career" goal after another. She was the salutatorian of her high school graduating class of more than 500 students. She graduated Phi Beta Kappa with a degree in special education from a prestigious private university. She earned national "Teacher of the Year" honors during only her fourth year of work. Then, intrigued by the field of psychiatric nursing, she returned to school to bolster her background in the basic sciences and entered nursing school. She was working as a staff nurse when she met Jim and planned to do graduate training in nursing.

Beverly was drawn to Jim by his intelligence and ambition—and his loneliness. He struck her as a man who had lived his life lost in his pursuit to become a physician. She also believed that Jim had not received his fair share of love and nurturing along the way. Beverly knew that she had much love to give, and Jim seemed to bask in the warmth of her attention.

This couple was very much in love and very much in agreement that, once they married, Beverly would probably quit her job and delay graduate training. They decided that one of them should be available as the "stress absorber" in their relationship during its early years and that Beverly was the person best suited for that role. Beverly was happy with this decision; she was ready for a break from her achievement-oriented lifestyle. Jim was ecstatic with this contract. His dreams of practicing medicine and having a loving wife to nurture and support him were apparently about to come true.

Like most medical couples, the Warrens began their marriage by negotiating a contract that worked wonderfully for both of them. This is an example of how early relationship contracting involves prioritizing and a division of roles and often means that one or both spouses have to put aspects of their "selves" on the shelf at least temporarily. A classic study of medical students and their wives reported that most wives of male medical students find fulfillment at first as facilitator of their mates' demanding career and stress absorber in the relationship.[3] Not surprisingly, this same study found that being married to a "stress absorber" helped relieve the burden of medical training.

Many medical couples actually share more time running their family during medical training than they will at any other time of their relationship. Recent research has shown that, as residents, more than 60 percent of physician-fathers tend to be involved in all facets of child care. As was already mentioned, most such couples assume that once training is over, the physician will *increase* time spent at home. What a disappointment it is when training ends and involvement in home and family life actually *decreases* for most physicians.

Renegotiating Your Relationship Contract

Medical couples like the Warrens run the risk that one or both of them will forget that they *each* have aspects of themselves that they agreed to downplay in order to create harmony during the initial stage of their relationship. As any relationship progresses, both partners experience a stirring to reclaim those aspects of their identities that were put on hold. This might require a major change in relationship teamwork.

Beverly and Jim Warren returned to counseling during the thirteenth year of their marriage. A self-diagnosed couple in trouble, they had been struggling for nine months to work out how they would make time and space for Beverly to return to nursing. She was now forty-two years old and was feeling a strong need to realize her own career ambitions. What Jim and Beverly had assumed would be a simple matter had become a relationship nightmare: They were questioning each other's loyalty and commitment and were locked into growing conflicts and fears. In short, the Warrens needed help renegotiating their relationship contract.

Growth in an intimate relationship depends on your ability to renegotiate cooperatively, lovingly, and periodically your relationship contract. None of us—no matter how dynamic we are—will be an exception to this rule.

Each of us changes as we accumulate life experiences. New experiences shape fresh "layers" of our personality, and maturity leads to new awareness of old layers of our personality that were not so obvious before. The more aware we become, the more compelled we are to be honest with ourselves and with each other. One result of the maturation process is that we only *truly* find out important information about ourselves and each other by marrying and hanging in there for the long haul.

Renegotiating the Obvious. Renegotiating your relationship contract often involves making obvious changes, some of which may be simple to implement and acceptable to both of you. For example, Beverly and Jim might have had no difficulty adjusting their schedules to make room for Beverly's return to graduate school or to her work as a nurse. In many ways, they might have made room in their life for Beverly to once again express those aspects of herself that had been put on the shelf during the initial stages of their marriage. Making such *obvious* changes in lifestyle might have gone quite smoothly for the Warrens if they had not stumbled into an unexpected wall blocking the smooth growth of their relationship.

Renegotiating the Not-So-Obvious. The Warrens hit the same wall that plagues most vital couples: distress about the not-so-obvious aspects of the relationship contract that *also* need to be renegotiated.

Beverly was supposed to be the nurturer of home and family, and Jim was the career-oriented physician in need of loving care. These roles were agreed upon early by Beverly and Jim.

But the Warrens experienced their own version of a universal quirk in marriage: the most complex aspects of relationship contracts are unspoken. One partner might secretly hope to change the other in a certain way. A nurturing caretaker who marries a hot-tempered bully hopes that love and nurturing will help the hot reactor calm down and deal differently with anger. Such unexpressed clauses in relationship contracts usually turn from hopes into expectations, which leads to significant marital tension.

Even more complicated are clauses that are unconscious. Here we are referring to the gut-level emotional and psychological needs that have never been soothed in past relationships, including (and often beginning) in our first family.

When these hopes turn into expectations, the stage is set for disappointment, distress, and disillusionment. What started out as a relationship that held the promise of ultimate happiness threatens to settle into what feels like the ultimate double-cross. It soon seems as though our partner's refusal to be how we need him or her to be is the reason for all of our pain—past and present.

Struggling to Renegotiate. The struggle to renegotiate the less-than-obvious parts of your contract are usually complicated and can fill your marriage with negative feelings—anxiety about how your relationship is turning out and anger that may be an exaggerated response to specific issues that you are facing.

After thirteen years of marriage, Beverly and Jim were living a life filled with responsibilities. Their days and weeks hummed with the activities of their daughters, aged nine and twelve. They enjoyed their beautiful home and vacation cottage but couldn't find time to maintain those residences. They scrambled to keep up with their burgeoning social life. Recently, they had also become the primary caretakers and source of financial support for Beverly's aging mother.

Jim was a senior partner in his growing orthopedic practice and was struggling to adjust to the demands and changes in the medical marketplace. He secretly worried about escalating overhead and diminished income.

Although she was not pursuing her profession, Beverly found herself exhausted by her daily schedule. The message on her car's bumper sticker resonated: "If a mother's place is in the home, then why am I always in this station wagon?"

These good people were each giving 100 percent, but were still having difficulty attending to the business of their life. Where in the world were they going to find the time and energy for Beverly's return to nursing or to graduate school?

Beverly was even more haunted by this question than Jim. She lay awake nights, facing a never-ending string of "what ifs": "What if I have to work afternoons or evenings? Who will cart the kids to their after-school lessons? What if I am working the second shift and Jim is on call? Will Jim be able to leave his office in the middle of the day if one of the kids gets sick and has to come home from school? I know that he won't be able to leave surgery, but I wonder if he will interrupt his office hours if need be. What if I end up having to work swing shifts? I can't even think about that.

"What about this house? Even with additional help, I know that I'll still be the one responsible for seeing that everything gets done."

Beverly was well aware of the complexity of the transition that faced them. Yet it felt like a supreme double-cross when Jim voiced his own reservations about the proposed change in lifestyle. At first, Jim's concerns were focused on practicalities and paralleled Beverly's own concerns: Who will chauffeur the children? What about emergency child-care needs? How was he supposed to suddenly make his demanding schedule more flexible?

The real trouble started when Beverly began to feel a familiar sense of irritation and hurt as she and Jim struggled with the issue. She began to feel that Jim was silently critical of her for disrupting their life with this midlife change of course. She accused him of having changed. He used to be a supportive and loving fan of hers. Now, by questioning her return to work, he seemed to have forgotten that she was just as competent as he.

At the same time, Jim accused Beverly of having changed. She used to thrive on loving and nurturing. Now she seemed hell-bent on proving that her career was just as important as his. Beverly and Jim soon struggled to an impasse.

The Underlying Pain. The issues underlying such an impasse almost always have to do with emotional needs of one or both spouses that are being frustrated, rather than soothed, by the current relationship contract. To resolve their impasse, Beverly and Jim needed to do four things: (1) become aware of their respective underlying issues, (2) learn to differentiate relationship issues from individual psychological struggles that signaled a need for growth, (3) correct the unrealistic expectations and maladaptive forms of communicating that were fueling their struggle to renegotiate their relationship contract, and (4) support each other. First, let's look at Beverly and Jim's underlying issues.

Despite her achievements, Beverly carried a deeply felt hurt: her father always paid more attention to the careers and accomplishments of her two brothers. He was of the old school and felt that a woman's place was in the home. Beverly recalled, "There I was, second in a class of 500, standing a good chance of winning an academic scholarship to a major university, and all my dad had to offer was the sage advice, 'You ought to take typing before you leave high school just in case you have to work as a secretary.'"

When she met Jim, his interest in, and validation of, her accomplishments appealed to her on a gut level. She felt as if she had finally found someone who would love her in a way that assuaged her deepest emotional needs.

Jim, on the other hand, felt that in Beverly he had found a solution to his own developmental pains. Beverly's interest in using her talents and energies to make a comfortable home and a loving family soothed him where he most hurt. Jim's own parents had divorced early in his life, and his mother's subsequent need to work outside their home left Jim alone much of the time.

"I was an only child who was home alone a lot. But I have nothing but love and admiration for my mother. She was gone simply because she had to work. It wasn't her fault. I thank God for her and for what she did for me.

"Still, I spent a lot of time alone. I was a 'latchkey' kid before the term was invented. I just don't want my kids to go through that.

"Look, I know that Beverly is a smart, talented woman. I know that if she had stayed in education, she'd have her doctorate now and would probably be a principal or an administrator or a college professor. If she

returns to nursing, she'll rise to the top—or wherever she wants to be—in that profession, too. But she didn't say that this is what she wanted to do with her life. We got married and had kids. If she planned to do this, I wish she would have told me. This wasn't the deal.

"At this point in our life, I don't see how we can do this without all of us going through a lot of pain. I love my life, starting with my family and my home, and I am not excited about having it turned upside down. If Beverly goes to work now, all of us are in for some hard changes. I know I need to be supportive of her, but what am I supposed to do about how I feel?

Gaining insight into these underlying concerns was helpful to the Warrens. Their compassion for each other increased as they saw each other grapple with these childhood issues. By learning why they were reacting to each other with such emotional urgency, they were able to dispel some of the fear that they were losing control of their relationship.

However, as Jim questioned the feasibility of his wife's return to her career, Beverly felt discounted and feared that her need to be acknowledged as a powerful person by the most important man in her life would not be met. The more Beverly reacted to this alarm by becoming preoccupied and upset, the more she fueled Jim's fears of being emotionally cut off from the most important woman in his life. The more alarmed Jim felt, the more critical he seemed to Beverly; the more alarmed Beverly felt, the more unavailable she seemed to Jim.

Like many couples, the Warrens gained intellectual insights into their dilemma, but their impasse continued. As their discomfort mushroomed, they settled into the power-struggle stage of marriage.

The Power Struggle

Any relationship that lasts long enough will eventually settle into one form or another of power struggle. Each partner tries to get the other to change enough to match their conscious and unconscious images and hopes.

Fuel for the Power Struggle. The power struggle is fueled by discomfort from several sources. First, life gets more complicated than anyone bargained for, and part of the complication seems to be your partner's refusal to be everything you need.

As explained by Gus Napier,

> Our failure to sustain this idealized union . . . reawakens in us a sense of ancient injury; our disappointment with ourselves and our mate reminds us of our disappointments with ourselves and our parents when we were children. Our mate becomes the "bad parent," while we feel like a "bad self." All the rage and hurt of those early years may then pour out into our marriage.[1(p14)]

Finally, the power struggle is fueled by discomfort that comes from the very essence of what was originally so attractive about your one true love—the fact that your partner in many ways embodied traits lurking in you unexpressed. Joining so closely with this person means encountering your own internal prohibitions against expressing certain thoughts, feelings, and ways of being. As stated by Harville Hendrix, "What first attracted you and momentarily liberated you, will eventually stir up what has been forbidden, causing you to squirm in discomfort."[2(p165)]

Power Struggling and TYABP. The power struggles we are referring to do not involve such superficial things as the television's remote control. Here we are referring to power struggles that are a threat to your very senses of well-being. Issues take on urgency; you feel compelled to change something *fundamental* about the other person.

The power struggle stage in a medical marriage can be significantly complicated if one (or both) partners is markedly Type A. The big bazookas of TYABP can lock couples into escalating combat as each tries to outdo the other in hardheaded, self-focused attempts to coerce an "I win" or an "I am back in control" outcome.

Once embroiled in a conflict of this sort, Type A's become so narrowly focused that they are not likely to relinquish control even when it is in their own best interest to do so. What's worse, Type A's also perceive compromising as being the same as losing.

If a sense of control is not soon restored, Type A's next react in a surprising fashion: they lapse into a state of withdrawal that belies their typically high-powered way of facing challenges. This withdrawal mimics a state of helplessness. The awkwardness and frustration of being helpless to regain control of something so important to them stirs a barrage of physiological stress reactions. The combination of helplessness and sympathetic nervous system supercharging can leave Type A's feeling as if they are powerful automobiles having the accelerator and brakes applied at once.

In our clinical work we have found that, in one way or another, misguided reactions to this stage of marriage are the most frequent underlying causes of divorce. It seems to be especially likely for those physicians who marry during the course of training. Approximately 50 percent of American medical students marry before graduation, and nearly 60 percent of such marriages end in divorce, compared to divorce rates of 40 to 50 percent for the general American population.[4]

The Stages of the Power Struggle. Regardless of who they are as individuals, couples progress through predictable stages of power struggling, which need to be anticipated.

First, they accuse each other. "You promised!"

This accusation can take many forms:

"You promised you would be the caretaker of our home and family, and now you want to leave us to go to work."

"You promised you would enjoy my family, and now all you do is criticize them."

"You promised you would slow down once you got out of residency, but now you're working more than ever."

Next, they lament, "You've changed."

"Why is this such a problem for you? You act surprised to know something that was the first thing I told you about myself. I just want to keep being who I have always been. You're *the one who's changed, not me."*

When neither of these strategies works to get the other person to change, couples resort to pleading, "For the sake of."

"For the sake of our marriage, why don't you slow this plan down."

"For the sake of our kids, why don't you stop this."

"For the sake of my career, you have *to get rid of this problem."*

"For God's sake, why don't you just shape up and become who I always thought you would become!"

The Pursuer-Distancer Dance

As the struggling continues, tensions mount in the relationship and erode intimacy. Many couples react with a strange form of teamwork that actually perpetuates marital problems: one partner assumes the role of pursuer, always seeking more contact, communication, resolution of conflict, and intimacy from the other. The other partner reflexively reacts with distancing. Distance may be maintained by showing lack of interest, by being fatigued, or by constantly being distracted or preoccupied with anything but the relationship. Some distancers literally exit; they stay away from the relationship, avoiding the pursuer by increasing hours spent at work, on the golf course, or in another relationship.

For many medical couples, the roles in this relationship dance become all too familiar. This dance also tends to be self-perpetuating: The more the pursuer pursues, the more the distancer distances. When the pursuer finally gets tired or fed up and withdraws, the distancer suddenly becomes interested. With renewed optimism, the couple may connect briefly, only to have the distancer back off, and the frustrating dance continues.

What fuels this pursuer-distancer dance is anxiety. On the one hand, there's anxiety about losing connection with that one true love and the parts of one's disowned self that are represented in that person. On the other hand, there's anxiety about getting too close to that same person and those same disowned traits. The pursuer-distancer pattern allows two people, each with their own conflicts about their split-off parts, to modulate the degree of contact they have with the living manifestation of their respective unexpressed selves—the other partner.

As the emotional tone of the marriage shifts in these negative ways, many couples settle into the next stage of the relationship journey—the dysfunctional communication pattern called *triangulation*.

Triangles

We said earlier that relationships tend to follow certain rules regardless of the players involved. One of them is that when two people are not getting along, they automatically divert their attention to something or someone else. Couples in conflict often avoid facing their most difficult relationship issues by focusing on a shared problem. Some people team up to worry about external stresses that affect their relationship. Some focus on a shared concern about another family member. Often the couple focuses on a specific problem being faced by one or both spouses (such as job pressures or a health problem). In any of its forms, this relationship pattern is called *triangulation* because the communication process can be depicted as a triangle.

Medical marriage and its inherent stresses predispose couples to develop communication triangles. Unless the partners learn to control this tendency, the relationship will suffer.

You will probably have to pause for only a moment to realize just how much the above statement applies to you. A medical couple's life fills with demands that take them away from each other *unless they fight to protect their connection.*

Like Beverly and Jim Warren, most medical couples spend the initial years of marriage cooperating to create a complicated lifestyle and learning to manage their stresses. In this sense, stress initially joins together most medical couples.

But when complex developmental hurdles appear, this same style of "teamwork" can lead any medical couple to avoid each other and to exacerbate tensions. The result is triangulation that erodes, rather than enhances, the relationship, for if you consistently attend to something or someone else *more* than each other, marital trouble is on the way.

Triangles, Work, and Medical Couples

We have never met a medical couple who did not have a convenient, ever-present diversion from their relationship tensions—work pressures. Excessive preoccupation with work can obviously *cause* relationship stress. But excessive involvement in work often seems to be a way of avoiding marital conflicts. As was mentioned before, Gabbard and Menninger have cautioned that many medical marriages progress from a "psychology of postponement" to a "psychology of avoidance." They state:

> The illusion of postponement hides a disturbing truth: that physicians actually *prefer* work to family life, that postponement is not so much delay as avoidance—avoidance of intimacy and marital involvement. Work becomes an effective defense against intimacy.[5]

Why does this happen? First, it is important to remember that, stress notwithstanding, most physicians still find their work quite satisfying. On the other hand, most physicians experience pronounced discomfort dealing with relationship dramas. Physicians tend to be scripted to please others. On the other hand, the demands of medical education and training, which typically last until age thirty, promote and reinforce in a physician a nonpersonalized style of relating to people. The result is a middle-aged man or woman who has well-honed role-related skills—like taking charge, staying logical in the heat of crisis, and maintaining emotional detachment despite high levels of stress. But skills for interpersonal intimacy are often lacking. Despite his or her overall power and competency, a physician may also harbor other psychological concerns that work *against* the ability to resolve marital conflict.

Research has repeatedly shown that, as a group, physicians tend to be perfectionistic and susceptible to self-doubt and guilt feelings, to harbor a chronic sense of emotional impoverishment, to have difficulties managing dependency and aggression, and to suffer a limited capacity for emotional expressiveness. As Gabbard and Menninger warned: "The language of feelings may be entirely alien, especially for the male physician."[5(p2380)]

So where is a physician embroiled in a growing power struggle with his or her pursuing mate to go? To work.

During these difficult stages of marriage, we are essentially told that we are not measuring up to the expectations of our one true love who claimed to know and accept us above all others. This criticism shakes us to our core. In addition, we begin seeing each other in a new, less-than-flattering light, *and* we are forced to accept the limits of our ability to change each other. This leaves even the most high-powered among us feeling wounded and impotent.

When both spouses are running from marital tensions, excessive work involvement can serve a defensive purpose. As one of the physicians in L. A. Gerber's *Married to Their Careers: Family Dilemmas in Doctors' Lives* so poignantly put it:

> "I really think that the reason I worked so hard at my practice, working to be special and needed, was so that I felt I wasn't alone."[6]

As focusing on work becomes the major refuge in the relationship, triangular patterns of communication become the habit, and the couple accumulates even more tension and drifts even further apart.

Reproducing Triangles

Communication triangles multiply rapidly. Any relationship stuck in one communication triangle is at risk of developing additional triangles.

Medical families that organize around a traditional division of marital roles often show a classic pattern of triangulation among three factions: the marital team, the husband's work, and the children. Here the physician-father becomes preoccupied with career, and the mother-wife becomes overly involved with the children. As they face stressful developmental stages (e.g., the children's adolescence), the triangulated family usually becomes more maladaptive. The relatively absent physician-father may begin to blame his wife for his own lack of closeness with his children. The children, already more involved with the mother, may become her confidants, thus perpetuating the triangulation.

In another version of this pattern, the parent who is relatively uninvolved in family life is idealized by the children, and the more involved parent becomes the scapegoat and feels insult being added to injury.

The case of Beverly and Jim Warren gives life to this concept.

As our counseling with Beverly and Jim continued, it became apparent that the process of triangulation was adding fuel to the fires in their marriage. The Warrens' triangles revolved around two factors: Jim's excessive work involvement and their twelve-year-old daughter, Sylvia. As Beverly explained it:

"I feel like a fool. I've spent my adulthood being a supportive partner for Jim, starting with my commitment to take up the slack that his work hours create in our family life. I've been a devoted 'physician's wife,' as I understood the needs of the role. I'm the one who attended every one of Sylvia's school plays, ball games, dance recitals. You name it, I was there. I spent my life in that station wagon, carting her and her friends all over creation. Now she decides that her daddy is 'Mr Wonderful Nurturing Parent of the Decade' and I am the 'Wicked Mother of the South.' I can't believe this! Kids! How can you guess what they will do next?

"But I'll tell you what I'm having an even harder time believing: Jim acts like he's loving this! I feel double-crossed. I want his support in dealing with Sylvia. I want him to say that what is happening in my relationship with Sylvia is natural, that it makes sense that Sylvia would take out her adolescent frustrations on me, given that I am the mother and the most convenient target for her young, hormonal raging. But no, he isn't saying any such thing. He's just quietly or not so quietly siding with Sylvia. It makes me furious! Our marriage is complicated enough

right now without Jim taking sides against me in dealing with Sylvia's sassy attitude.

"As I was telling my sister the other day, I know good and well what he's doing. He's angry with me because I'm not so 'hot to trot' under the sheets with him anymore in the middle of the night—after I have hardly seen him all week. He has pinned this rap on me, accusing me of being 'unnurturing.' He acts like my wanting to go back to school or to work is 'unnurturing.' He's even acting like our daughter's adolescence is due to the fact that I am 'unnurturing.' If I hear that word one more time, I'll scream. My God, I am screaming! I'm fed up with this mess!

"Maybe my sister was right in the first place. You know, she never really liked Jim. She never liked the idea of my marrying a man who wanted me to give up my career. What am I going to do?"

At this point, Beverly and Jim's family life was filled with communication triangles. Jim and his daughter were joined in a way that excluded Beverly, and Beverly and her sister were joined in a triangle that excluded Jim.

Controlling the Triangles

Triangles are never solutions to relationship problems; they only complicate matters. The key to controlling triangulation is to take care of the business brewing in the relationship that is spawning triangles. For example, the mess that developed in the Warren family would never have cleared unless Beverly and Jim were willing to deal directly with *each other* about their concerns (which, fortunately, they were).

We are not saying that marital harmony is a cure-all. No matter how happily married you are, adolescents will still struggle with their parents, or an in-law may not approve of your spouse, or any number of the stresses and disappointments of real life may cause problems. But we *are* saying that the relationship that contains the most shared information will be the relationship that is most intimate.

Relationship teamwork is your most powerful lever in dealing with stressful times, including the stresses of problem relationships *within* your family. Teamwork does not require that you agree on everything. In fact, as we explored their situation further, we found that Jim had a number of valid criticisms about how Beverly was parenting their daughter. In the heat of the triangle, Beverly was reflexively reacting to Sylvia with criticism, often inappropriately so.

But Jim needed to convey this information in a loving way *within the privacy of his marriage,* not in a gossiping way in collusion with his daughter. Similarly, Beverly harbored many valid points of criticism about Jim's way of reacting to their conflicts. But she needed to convey these *to her husband,* not to her sister.

The Danger of Triangles

A final word about communication triangles is in order. We need to emphasize that triangulation is more than uncomfortable; it is also dangerous.

Research has shown that a child's physiological stress reactions elevate when the child is drawn into triangulation between troubled parents.[7] Because a relationship triangle is usually a web filled with conflicts of loyalty, anyone—child or adult—caught in this web is likely to react with alarm felt on both emotional *and* physical levels. This stress can actually lead to physical illness.

Furthermore, as distance grows in a relationship locked in triangulation and as the triangles multiply, new, even more complex conflicts of loyalty develop. For example, once Beverly began gossiping about her marriage to her sister, she had a new problem on her hands: now her closeness with her sister revolved around sharing a growing disapproval of her husband. How would she deal with this? To whom would she be more loyal? Who would be her main confidant and most intimate partner: her husband or her sister? Furthermore, how would she resolve the dilemma of wanting intimate connections with *both* these important people while living in the double bind of knowing that if she moved closer to one of them, she would distance herself from the other?

It is not far-fetched to propose that, given this situation, both Beverly and Jim were also at risk of developing even more complicated alliances outside their marriage. This is a nice way of saying that triangulation is often the stuff of which extramarital affairs are made.

For Beverly and Jim Warren, what started out as a need to renegotiate certain parts of their relationship contract in order to make roc-n for Beverly's career ended up being a mass of reactions and counterreactions that shook their relationship to its very core.

An authentic, lasting romance cannot be constructed on the shifting psychological sands at the foundation of the "one true love" stage of romance. The one-true-love phenomenon does serve an important purpose: It allows us to feel safe enough to fall in love. But remember, this stage largely has to do with our individual struggles with the split-off parts of ourselves that we see manifested in our partner and that we hope our partner will soothe. Struggling with another person about these issues is a way of creating a new and more productive struggle with *our own* split-off parts. In this sense, the "power struggle" stage of marriage, too, serves a crucial, positive purpose. These struggles do *not* mean that your marriage is dying. Quite the contrary; they are signs of growth.

As Harville Hendrix so eloquently states:

> The power struggle, like romantic love, is another way station en route to
> the real thing. . . . It is supposed to happen. . . . It is not even a negative

indicator, but a sure sign that we are with the right person for our maximum potential growth—if we handle it correctly.[2(p231)]

References

1. Napier A. *The Fragile Bond: In Search of an Equal, Intimate and Enduring Marriage.* New York, NY: Harper & Row;1988:225.
2. Hendrix H. *Keeping the Love You Find: A Guide for Singles.* New York, NY: Pocket Books; 1992:21.
3. Combs RH, Fawzy FI. The effect of marital status on stress in medical school. *Am J Psychiatry.* 1982;139:1490-1493.
4. Marchand WR, Palmer CA, Gutmann L, Brogan WC. Medical student impairment: a review of the literature. *W Va Med J.* 1985;81:244-248.
5. Gabbard GO, Menninger RW. The psychology of postponement in the medical marriage. *JAMA.* 1989;261:2378-2381.
6. Gerber LA. *Married to Their Careers: Family Dilemmas in Doctors' Lives.* New York, NY: Tavistock; 1983.
7. Minuchin S, Rosman B, Baker L. *Psychosomatic Families: Anorexia Nervosa in Context.* Cambridge, Mass: Harvard University Press; 1978.

Whom Are You Going to Choose? Declaring Your Loyalty as You Work Through Disillusionment

When you see through love's illusions, there lies the danger. And your perfect lover just looks like a perfect fool.

—Jackson Browne, *"Fountain of Sorrow"*

So now it is down in black and white: there is no doubt that marriage changes relationships, often in the very ways that you dread. No matter how mature you are, how experienced at love and romance you become, or how long you date (or live together) before you marry, one thing is certain: You will only *really* get to know each other when married.

It *is* possible to have healthy and happy partnerships that never progress to marriage. But the operative word in the preceding sentence is "progress."

We believe that you continue to progress to new levels of self-discovery and relationship growth only if you marry and channel your energies into keeping your relationship alive. And we are not alone in this conviction. Internationally, growing attention is being paid to the "save marriage" movement.

Even with all of its inherent struggles, we believe in marriage. Today, more than ever, people need the enduring, intimate connection that can only come from marriage. We are social beings. As such, we define and discover certain essential aspects of our selves only within relationships. The most intense, penetrating, stimulating, and hopefully nurturing social context is a long-term marriage, one that is unlimited in its height, breadth, and depth.

In a nutshell, we believe that marriage complicates and enhances growth. It raises the ceiling of self-knowledge *and* lowers its floor into deeper intrapsychic terrain for each spouse and for the relationship.

The Negative Side of Marriage

Contrary to many contemporary authors who promote the message that marriages should endure at all costs, we believe that some marriages need to be put to rest. Relationships that are toxic rather than nurturing and affirming need to either change for the better or end.

Managing your emotional and physical health is serious business, and you need a partner who is willing to help you in this regard. Ohio State University researcher Janice Kiecolt-Glaser demonstrated how women suffer negative consequences in their autoimmune system functioning following marital conflict.[1] And University of Washington researcher John Gottman demonstrated how men experience exaggerated cardiovascular and other autonomically driven stress reactions during conflictual marital interchanges.[2]

Medical couples sometimes face the choice to either become more authentically caring or end their relationship.

Of course, we remind them that divorce comes at considerable emotional and financial cost to all involved. It pains us that so many people rush off to divorce court in a self-focused frenzy fueled by misguided motives. For some, the catalyst is the semi-brain-damaged way of thinking that occurs during infatuation with a new "one true love." Others are demoralized rather than challenged by the developmental struggles they are facing in their marriage. Still others are caught up in an urgent quest for some vaguely defined thing that they think exists only outside their marriage. Rather than work on their marriage or themselves, they evade disillusionment by fleeing in general.

When you face difficult times in your marriage, our advice to you is try your best to address the issues that are frustrating you. Instead of growing wise as you leave your marriage, and applying that wisdom to a new chapter of your life, why not get wise enough to *keep your marriage's intimacy factor* larger than any issues that face you?

What if this simply does not work to lessen the toxicity of your relationship? As passionately as we believe in marriage, we also believe that living in a toxic relationship is more than costly; it is destructive. Here's an example of a marriage that needed to either get more caring or end.

Edie and Simon

We once counseled a physician named Edie who had endured repeated and profound sexual abuse by her father and various other male authority figures throughout her childhood and early adolescence. Eventually, she married Simon, a man who promised to be her nurturing rescuer, who seemed interested in her for reasons that had to do with love, not sexual exploitation. In the seeming safety of this marriage, Edie came alive with the excitement of getting physically and emotionally healthy. She underwent years of psychotherapy and committed herself to "reparenting" herself, starting with a vow to take more loving care of her physical self.

In many ways, Simon was the original and most enduring fan of Edie's personal growth. He was the first person to encourage her to seek therapy. Throughout her initial years of treatment, Simon nurtured Edie when she floundered, always reassuring her of his continued love and support. Simon was also an ideal physician's husband. Throughout Edie's years of training, he took up the slack at home. He encouraged and bolstered Edie when her shaky self-esteem led her to doubt herself. Simon took pride in Edie. But in a crucial area this couple settled into a way of interacting that actually hurt rather than helped Edie's efforts to heal her deepest wounds.

Due to his own insecurities about whether or not he was truly lovable, Simon eventually began to invalidate the "new" Edie. He seemed threatened by having to keep up with a mature, healthy, vibrant wife. At first, his invalidation took the form of teasing her about her ever-changing versions of herself. Soon he started accusing her in a shaming way of "trying to be something you read about in books; not real and not really you."

Such chiding hurt and confused Edie. But Simon's eventual way of dealing with their sexual relationship went beyond confusing; it became toxic to Edie's fundamental well-being. Ostensibly due to her hang-ups, for many years Edie and Simon avoided sexual intercourse, settling for self-stimulation while lying next to each other. Now Edie was ready to incorporate her sexuality into the fold of her sense of self. She invited her husband to experiment with her in learning to have what she believed to be "normal" sex—sex that involved loving intercourse.

But here, too, Edie's need for validation as a growing individual collided with her husband's refusal to acknowledge and take responsibility for his own issues. Simon refused "normal" sex, stating that he preferred the intense stimulation that came from masturbating and ejaculating onto Edie as she watched him enjoy his orgasm.

To even an untrained eye, the problem with Edie's participation in this form of sex was obvious. To Edie, this no longer felt like sex "play" but like once again being sexually abused. This sexual impasse characterized much about the spirit of Edie and Simon's marriage. To Edie, remaining in this marriage would be to choose continued abuse. The thought of doing so violated her commitment to reparent herself.

Aware of the seriousness of the dilemma, Edie dragged Simon into counseling with us. Over the course of several months of therapy, Simon demonstrated his understanding of how their marriage was replicating a traumatic process for Edie, but he steadfastly refused to change. Through his self-centered behavior, Simon underscored a major clause that always existed in their relationship contract: "Given that I am willing to accept you, even as flawed as you are from all of the abuse you have been through, you owe me whatever I want."

Once all of the above was made clear, Edie and her husband faced a choice. Either both of them would muster the courage it would take to grow in a healthy direction, or they would separate.

Ambivalently, but with integrity and compassion, Edie ended their marriage, motivated by the insight that to continue in the relationship was to choose a toxic, maladaptive life that would aggravate rather than heal her most serious psychological wounds.

Crisis and Disillusionment in Marriage

It is easier to decide whether or not to stay in a marriage when the quality of the relationship is clear: clearly wonderful (so stay married!) or clearly abusive (so get out!). This call is easy to make when considering someone *else's* marriage.

More difficult is deciding what to do when your distress is due to disillusionment, not abuse. In an article that addressed stress and burnout in the medical profession, Jack McCue cautioned that fleeing from disillusionment can lead to misguided attempts at solutions, including making a drastic career change or trading one marital partner for another.[3]

> A retreat to the quiet life in a small town is more likely to move one's career discontents to that small town than to resolve them. Likewise, the physician who thinks that an unhappy home life is making his job unpleasant is missing the obvious; his unhappiness is affecting both his marriage and work, and changing spouses won't make medicine more enjoyable.[3(p16)]

What should you do when you wake up and find yourself waist-deep in the disillusionment stage of marriage? This is *the* question that medical couples most often bring into our offices. For the most part, our clients are not people who are battling horrible demons, like the residuals of profound childhood abuse. Our clients are typically people in distress. Often theirs is a distress born of disillusionment about the struggles that fill their lives, both as individuals and as a couple.

Now we turn to another universal factor that affects marriage and that increases the risk of settling into disillusionment: crisis. By crisis we mean those times when you are faced with problems that you seem incapable of resolving. These are times when your stresses seem to outweigh your resources. Crisis happens when something threatens your stability—as an individual, couple, or family—and you feel incapable of resolving it.

From this perspective, the power-struggle and disillusionment stages of marriage are filled with crises. Both stages involve facing what is threatening and difficult to control. Both stir our deepest ambivalence. In addition, crisis makes many people project blame and displace anger; we decide that the *real* source of our distress is a tangible, definable entity—*our partner.*

We have no doubt that, for many medical couples, this misguided way of responding to crisis is what leads to divorce. Few life experiences meet the defining criteria of crisis as fully as undergoing medical training.

When medical students enter the clinical years of training, they face long absences from home, sleep deprivation, and the anxiety of caring for sick and dying people before becoming truly competent in the practice of medicine. Their spouses also face a crisis—living with preoccupied, fatigued, and distressed partners.

In this situation, a spouse may refuse to acknowledge that the medical student is now unavailable and alter his or her daily routine accordingly. Meals are prepared and social events scheduled, all based on the fantasy that the medical student will show up. Some spouses even resort to spending hours in a parked car outside the medical center, harboring the delusion that the loved one will soon appear.

At first, the medical student may fuel such denial with unrealistic optimism regarding his or her ability to control his or her work schedule. But eventually, anger and despair set in for such couples. The spouse may become depressed, overcome by feelings of loneliness and unexpressed anger. Daily routines are abandoned, and disorganization rules the household.[4]

The spouse then channels his or her energies into activities outside the relationship. Due to his or her new commitments (new friends, a return to school, a child to care for), the spouse may not be available on the rare occasions that the medical student is, which fuels even more frustration and anger.

The result? *Both* partners drift into a sense of detachment. A new contract is negotiated that specifies more distance and less intimacy.

This process is fueled by dynamics that are similar to those described in the previous chapter's discussion of power struggling in marriage. Two rather shaky layers have now been added to the foundation of the medical marriage: the impasses that come with power struggling and disillusionment.

Disillusionment heightens as crises are encountered. However, here, too, we have an optimistic message about marriage: Crisis is an opportunity to grow.

Facing a crisis can be a turning point in any long-term relationship. When we face a crisis, we are forced to choose to move either closer or farther apart. Whether or not a specific crisis (or the power struggle or disillusionment stages of marriage) does permanent damage to your romance depends on what you do next. The case of Jim and Beverly Warren demonstrated how rapidly a relationship in crisis can settle into patterns that guarantee distance and damage intimacy. The case of the Warrens also underscores a warning that all couples are wise to heed: You are at particular risk of settling into marital disillusionment when you face major transitions in your life.

In the following pages, we describe a number of common crises faced by couples that may contribute to disillusionment. Some are inevitable developmental passages (like boredom and staleness); they come with the natural progression of life. Others, like extramarital affairs, are crises that can be avoided.

Use the following descriptions to take the temperature of your relationship. Let these descriptions form a road map for charting your past and anticipating potential potholes in your future. Note which hurdles you have already cleared, what you are now facing, and what might lie ahead for you.

Crisis 1: When One of You Is Ready to Change the Definition of Your Relationship and the Other Is Not

How do you define your relationship? This is a crucial question. Whether you have just met or have been together for many years, your degree of agreement or disagreement on this matter will have a clear effect on the quality of your relationship. Couples get into predictable conflict when they fail to agree on a definition of the state of their union—and when one member is more ready than the other to redefine the relationship.

We are not referring to those relationship-redefining times when you face some transition that requires an intense but limited period of cooperation, like having a new house built. Although such times are indeed stressful, couples are seldom confused about how to cope with this tangible kind of stress. They may get tired and vexed, but not confused.

Our concern here is what happens when you face threats to the status quo of your relationship. Such threats can shock you into awareness of your differences and shake the relationship to its core.

For example, we once counseled a couple who came to us in a crisis that began when the husband, an internist, was offered the opportunity to enter private practice in his native state of New York. When he received the job offer, he rushed home to share the good news with his wife. He was thrilled to finally get the chance to move back home, close to his extended family. Much to his surprise, his wife declared herself a dyed-in-the-wool North Carolinian and refused to even consider living elsewhere. The implications of her response were tremendously unsettling.

Did this mean that living in North Carolina was more important to the wife than her husband's career or his desire to be closer to his extended family? On the other hand, did this man's own career and family needs mean more than his wife's desire to remain in *her* own familiar territory?

What about the future? If he remained married to her, would he have to give up the dream of someday living closer to his extended family?

When couples begin defining their relationship out loud, sometimes their words paint a picture of incompatibility. Their life plans may not match. As another of our clients explained: "My husband wants to live his life in a way that gets him closer to the country club. I want to live my life in a way that gets me closer to the country." At last contact, these two were happily divorced. She was living on 15 acres of land in a rented farmhouse, and he was remarried to a woman who thrived on the social interplay of their cosmopolitan lifestyle.

More often, a threat to the status quo is due to differences in timing, pacing, and respective levels of satisfaction with things as they are. One partner is ready to move on to the next stage of relationship growth before the other one is ready to deal with the changes that will come with the transition. Some people are happy just to keep things the way they are in the relationship. Their needs are being met, so why mess with the status quo? Many hesitate out of fear of what might be lost—freedom, autonomy, control or power in the relationship—if the change is made.

On the one hand, each decision takes you closer to your partner. On the other hand, each involves entering uncharted territory, a prospect that carries with it the threat of losing some valued part of the way things are and of becoming more vulnerable to each other. These decisions are usually posed as questions that must be answered in the course of any relationship.

- Do you want to have a relationship that excludes becoming romantically or sexually involved with other people?
- Do you want to live together?
- Do you want to begin discussing marriage?
- Do you want to plan to get married?
- Do you want to pool your money?
- Are you willing to move emotionally further from certain people and closer to others for the sake of maintaining harmony in your relationship?
- Do you want to become parents?

This last question takes us to discussion of the next crisis faced by many couples.

Crisis 2: When New Members Are Added to Your Family

One of the most stressful times in any marriage is during the early childbearing and child-rearing years. The incidence of divorce during the marriage life cycle typically spikes during the years of parenting toddler-aged children. Becoming parents takes your relationship into totally new territory that is filled with both opportunities to create a meaningful life together and novel forms of stress.

No matter how vigorous you are, parenting will tap your stress reserves and stir your vulnerabilities. For most high-powered couples, having a child yields greater intimacy, trust, respect, and love for each other. However, here, too, predictable hurdles need to be cleared in order to grow as a couple.

A rule of group dynamics is that two-person systems experience tremendous tensions when they change into three-person systems. This, of course, makes sense: "Two's company; three's a crowd" and other such adages remind us of truths many medical couples know but are surprised to find out applies to *them*. No matter how deeply in love a couple is, once a baby comes, the husband will be (relatively) left out of the intimate relationship between wife and infant, at least for a period of time.

This is often a profound experience for a medical couple. Perhaps for the first time in the history of this intense relationship, admiration and facilitation of the husband's life are not the primary agenda. A new love affair and preoccupying concern have entered the marriage.

We are not saying that men cannot or should not be intimately involved in parenting their infant children, or that new parents automatically lose the romance in their marriage. Quite the contrary: We spend much of our professional lives helping men overcome their shyness and awkwardness about declaring themselves first-string players in family life. We spend another major chunk of our professional time helping couples understand that marriage can remain a passionate, intimate affair throughout their life.

We are simply stating what we believe to be a fact no matter how politically sensitive or psychologically skillful and healthy we become: During infancy and early childhood, the baby bonds first and most intensely with the mother, not the father.

Our own experience is a case in point. When Mary and I married, we planned to start a family immediately. One of the most romantic parts of our courtship was talking and daydreaming about how we would be as parents. We went into marriage and parenthood with the commitment to orchestrate our life so that I shared much of the parenting of our children, especially during their earliest years. This was due to our shared passion to parent.

Our dreams came true. Our daughter Rebecca was born nine and one-half months after our wedding, and two and one-half years later, Julia blessed us with her presence.

Because we are in private practice, Mary and I have always had the freedom to orchestrate our work schedules to our liking. During the early days of our family, we arranged our schedules to allow a true sharing of responsibilities for our children. I loaded three days with work and freed Tuesday and Thursday afternoons and every Friday to be home, caring for Rebecca and Julia. My head and heart are filled with memories of those days with my girls. To ensure their bonding with me during infancy, I often held them against my bare chest, loving that skin-to-skin contact. I fed them, bathed them, rocked them, loved them, and got to know them.

When they were both toddlers, Rebecca, Julia, and I spent our afternoons in beautiful Old Salem, a restored village in our hometown. I arranged *Kindermusik* lessons for each of them on alternating afternoons. While one attended her lesson, the other and I strolled around, played games, talked, and got a treat. I often worried about the "lost income" that resulted from spending this much time with my girls, but I consoled myself—and got loving consolation from Mary—with the reminder that this was money well spent.

Those were halcyon days for me. Unlike so many fathers whom I counseled, I knew that my children knew me and bonded with me from the beginning of their lives.

That was one aspect of what was happening during the early stages of our family. Another was that I was ready to claim periods of space from our children far sooner than Mary. I loved all the family togetherness, but I wanted romance and courtship, too. I remember tensions between Mary and me about our differences here. I just could not understand why, once the kids were beyond breastfeeding and well acquainted with our loving babysitter, Mary was still ambivalent about periodically going away for 24 or 36 hours of solitude and romance.

But ambivalent she was, caught in a bind of missing time alone with me and yet reluctant to leave our babies. Even though I understood it logically, Mary's ambivalence still felt like a barrier between us. I did not understand why I felt clearer and more comfortable about the psychological boundaries that separated me from our girls and delineated our romance from the coparenting part of our marriage. I could more comfortably disengage from our children for what I considered to be relatively brief periods of time. I knew that I loved them and cared for them as much as Mary did, so why was I ready to break away sooner than she? Was it that I loved Mary more than she loved me? Was it just that I was an insensitive man?

I got a glimpse of the answer on one rainy Saturday afternoon when Rebecca and Julia were five and three years old, respectively. Rebecca had a cold, and in order to get her to rest, we all decided to take naps. Of course, because she did not feel well, Rebecca got to sleep with her "Mommy." That left me and three-year-old Julia to snuggle in her bed.

As we lay there trying to get settled, Julia tickling the edge of her blanket and looking at me with her big, sleepy eyes, I was waxing semipoetically to myself about my little girl when she said, "My Daddy, would it hurt your feelings if I went to sleep with Mommy and Becca?"

(What!) "No, of course not." *(Calmly)* "Do you want to go sleep with your Mommy?"

(Sleepily, apologetically nodding her head)

"Well, that's okay. Little girls like to sleep with their mommies. But let me ask you something, Juice. What do you feel when you take a nap with Mom?"

"I don't know. Snuggly and good, I guess."

"That's nice. It does feel good to snuggle with your mom, doesn't it? *(Pause)* You can go sleep with Mommy. But before you go, let me ask you one more thing: What do you feel when you take a nap with your daddy?"

My humbling then came. Julia thought for a moment—but only for a moment. Then, my little Julia—the same child who looks like me, the same one whom I rocked bare-chested throughout her infancy, the same one for whom I "lost" thousands of dollars in income to take to music lessons on Tuesday and Thursday afternoons—this beautiful child, looked straight into my eyes and said the words: "Mild to medium."

Mild to medium?

I swear to you, that's what my daughter matter-of-factly said.

As Julia's words echoed in my head and she waddled toward her Mommy's loving arms, leaving me alone, sprawled out on her lace-edged canopy bed, I remember feeling humbled, amused, and—above all else—sort of in awe.

Mary and the children really did have something going on that excluded me. How ironic that in this most important arena of my life—my relationships with my wife and daughters—I had to settle for working hard to occupy a position on the sidelines. I was a valued substitute, but I was not really a first-string player.

In true manly form, I decided to take my high-powered self down to my study and do some paperwork.

We seldom meet a father who cannot relate to this story. If you don't go into parenthood humble, knowing that something powerful and mysterious will exist between mother and child, you will soon be taught that lesson. Many men have difficulty with this abrupt shift into sharing their wives' love and attention with another. Their wives' bonding with their babies creates a narcissistic wound; they feel abandoned or left out. In response, some men flee: into withdrawal, into work, or, worse yet, into relationships outside the marriage. Others strike out, quietly expressing their narcissistic rage over the "abandonment" by their one true love.

Women themselves are not immune to narcissistic wounding during this stage of marriage. A new mother may begin to resent the attention that her usually absent physician-husband showers on their children. She may feel rejected now that he can find time and energy to be such a nurturing father. Why hadn't he managed to find time and energy for her?

In addition, many new mothers are in conflict about their newly forming relationship with their baby. Such stirrings can take various forms. Some new mothers feel vulnerable and afraid, not sure that they are ready for motherhood. Some feel sadness or joy as they remember how they were mothered. Some ruminate over what aspects of their high-powered life will need to be compromised in order to be a good mother. Psychiatrist Michael Myers cautions that such conflicts are especially likely for female physicians, many of whom entered marriage ambivalent about the nurturing, domestic sides of themselves.[5]

Physician or not, damage is done to marital trust and intimacy when a woman looks around and finds her husband gone—literally or figuratively. The stress and disappointment that then occur during this early stage of marriage can end the relationship or cause wounds that last a lifetime.

On the other hand, this is the stage of marriage that welds most couples together. They reach higher levels of intimacy and deeper levels of trust as they clear hurdles that are unique to the experiences of coparenting.

Having children creates a double bind for most parents: The stresses of parenting change your life and marriage in ways that you may not enjoy on a given day. This dissatisfaction might lead you to wonder what life would be like if you ended your marriage. On the other hand, once children are part of your marriage, your commitment to each other deepens. The relationship becomes a richer and more meaningful place where something magical and identity-forming is happening for each of you. Fantasies of leaving the marriage in order to relieve the stresses of the relationship now get tempered with profound feelings of loss when you imagine disrupting your family. Your role in your family—however bittersweet it might seem on a given afternoon—becomes an integral and meaningful aspect of your identity.

Another anecdote from our marriage: Like many high-powered couples, we started our relationship with a clear warning to each other: "Treat me right or I'm gone!" As our home and hearts filled with those babies and all that came with them, this shared machismo dwindled with each passing day. When our girls were toddlers, we remember a conversation that went something like this: "You know that 'treat me right or I'm gone' business? I want to change the deal. Here's what I have to say to you now: 'Please, please, *please*, don't do anything bad to me! No matter what you do, I'm still going to be here tomorrow. So stay nice.' We used to be married; now we are Married!"

Crisis 3: Extramarital Affairs

Whether you get "caught" or not, an extramarital affair will change your marriage at least temporarily, often permanently. The trauma of an affair affects the trust and intimacy of both spouses.

If you are the "innocent" spouse, knowledge of your partner's affair disrupts your trust. Intimacy is eroded by anger, embarrassment, confusion, and sadness. You become obsessed with how the affair occurred, where it took place, and exactly what transpired between your partner and the other person. Feeling that you have been violated is perhaps the most difficult part of this trauma. As one woman put it after learning of her husband's affair: "I feel like someone broke into my home and went through my personal things. I feel like I've been violated, like I've been raped."

If you are the person who had the affair, your guilt, anxiety, or conflict of loyalties is likely to erode marital intimacy. In order to keep an affair secret, you must distance yourself from your partner. Interestingly, most people who have affairs actually feel that they are reacting to disillusionment in the marriage that was originally caused by the *other* spouse's disloyalty. They often report that they were the first in the marriage to feel abandoned. Basically, many people describe what was actually a period of triangulation preceding the affair. They claim that the affair resulted because of vulnerability they felt due to their mate's overinvolvement in work, in the lives of their children, or an extended family, their community, church, or friends—something or someone other than the marriage.

Affairs signal a marriage in need of healing from *both* sides. We have worked with couples and individuals who have had every kind of affair imaginable. When people become convinced that they need a change, they become infinitely creative in their ability to flirt with danger and inexhaustible in their willingness to take risks. Affairs run the gamut from impulsive to well-planned, responsibly negotiated decisions to have sexual relationships outside their marriage.

Our award for the most impulsive (and foolishly dangerous) affair goes to a woman who engaged in a fifteen-minute "roll on the floor" (her words) with her brother-in-law while her husband (the brother of the other party rolling on the floor) napped on the couch in the *same* room.

Our award for the most well-thought-out, sensitively orchestrated affair goes to two married couples who came to counseling together to make sure that everyone was communicating fully and clearly about what they *really* wanted and how they *really* felt about their proposed mate swapping. These same couples continued counseling for over a year in an effort to ensure that no one got hurt by what they collectively reasoned was "a sensible expansion of the unnecessary notion that happy marriage requires monogamy" (their words).

We have learned a universal lesson from these folks and from the thousands of other people we have counseled regarding affairs: If you have an affair, you can almost be guaranteed that the affair will damage—if not end—your marriage. We have yet to meet a couple who proved to be an exception to this statement.

We hasten to add that we *have* counseled hundreds of couples who survived the psychological storms of an affair (or affairs) and who actually grew more healthy and intimate in the aftermath. Many couples respond sensibly to trauma once it is over. They recognize that an affair signals a need to draw a line that separates the way they have heretofore operated from the way they will *now* deal with themselves and each other.

These couples ended the affairs and worked to heal from the trauma. The affair killed the old marriage. The affair ended. The couple once again chose each other. And then they cooperated in creating a "new" relationship.

Crisis 4: Boredom and Staleness

People often seek marriage counseling out of fear that they are heading toward divorce. The fear is sometimes based on a trauma that has severely damaged the marriage: an affair, substance abuse by one partner, or physical abuse, for example. But more often, our clients who fear they may be headed for divorce have not experienced any specific trauma. The most frequent reason that people seek our marriage counseling is that their passion and romance have died. Again, our clients put it succinctly:

David, husband of an internist: *"Is marriage supposed to be about sameness and routine even in the ways we make love?"*

Becky, wife of a radiologist: *"Is it just a part of growing up? Does that wonderful boyfriend-girlfriend action that used to survive even the stormiest times between us just go away as the years go on?"*

Harold, a rheumatologist: *"Does any couple really continue to discover new and different things about each other? How do you stay interested in someone once their 'mystery' is gone?"*

We privately joke that everything we know about life that is worth knowing we have learned from our clients. We are fortunate to have a practice that affords us opportunities to work with people who are thriving as well as with people who are suffering. From such clients—and our personal experience—we have learned to believe in the possibility of maintaining passion throughout the course of marriage.

Even the most passionate couples periodically face boredom and staleness in their marriage. Couples who do not enjoy a high level of romantic love often have an unrealistic impression of "all those other couples" who seem so comfortable in their romance. The stale couples tend to think that the couples who are "still crazy in love after all these years" just naturally "have it made." Maybe there are indeed some relationships that are so filled with reciprocating hormone storms that their collective biology overrides every other facet of relationship development.

More likely, however, no relationship remains romantic "naturally." Couples keep their romance going by working at it.

Perhaps even more important, thriving couples avoid staleness and boredom by keeping their friendship growing. The California Divorce Mediation Project is generally considered by experts in the field as one of the most outstanding studies of subjectively reported reasons for divorcing. It clearly documented that the majority of couples state that their reason for divorcing was essentially a loss of friendship.[2] On the other hand, as will be discussed in our chapter on preparing for retirement, couples who thrive during their second half of marriage point to their sustained or renewed friendship as being the most important factor determining their marital happiness.

Crisis 5: Career Crises

One guaranteed way to change your life is to face a career crisis, either your own or your partner's. Major career transitions—good or bad—run the risk of affecting more than your family income. Such changes can also affect marital teamwork and catapult you into disillusionment.

For contemporary medical couples, career crises come in many flavors: stress overload from career changes, burnout, unexpected job loss, struggles over whose career will take precedence in determining such factors as choosing a place to live or orchestrating daily life, simple boredom, and threats of or actual malpractice suits, to name a few possibilities.

This last factor is a concern for many medical couples. Statistics available from the American Medical Association's Socioeconomic Monitoring System indicate that, from 1985 to 1997, the incidence of malpractice suits filed against physicians declined significantly from 10.2 claims per 100 physicians in 1985 to the 1997 figure of 6.3 claims per 100 physicians. However, this same report emphasized a sobering fact: Fully 39.3 percent of all physicians experience at least one malpractice claim during their careers. Over 60 percent of all obstetricians/gynecologists and over half of surgeons have had at least one claim in their careers.[6]

The trauma of being targeted by such litigation is well documented and has recently been labeled malpractice stress syndrome.[7] For both spouses, being sued often leads to depression, anger, tension, frustration, irritability, insomnia, fatigue, somatic aches and pains, social withdrawal, guilt, shame, and denial. In addition, the disillusionment that comes with being sued leads many physicians into early retirement or a career shift.

While career crises can occur at any stage of life, questioning your career status is a predictable part of (and sometimes begins) midlife questioning. Once you have established a career, the thrill of working in that profession dies out. People often report feeling trapped, spending over one third of their lives in jobs that are no longer fulfilling. At a time in life when most people feel compelled to push for greater authenticity, they feel handcuffed to a job that has lost its meaning.

This is a situation fraught with traps. The spouse of the person in career crisis becomes anxious about the implications of the crisis. Frightening questions may fill the spouse's quiet reflections:

"What is this *really* all about?"

"What if my partner asks me to relocate or change how we are living in some major way?"

"Maybe he is just making a mountain out of a mole hill."

"I want to be supportive, but I'm not sure what I'm supporting. Maybe she just needs to 'bite the bullet' and hang in there. No one has a career that is always fulfilling—do they?"

The marital traps can multiply as the person going through the career crisis becomes preoccupied with ambivalence and self-questioning. "Maybe I just need to grow up and stop complaining. After all, I *am* making good money. On the other hand, I can't remember the last time I let *my* needs come first. Maybe it's time to have the guts to make a move."

In trying to defend oneself against the pain and confusion of this crisis, people often begin thinking in ways that can complicate their marriage.

"I don't know what to do. I'm miserable in this job but handcuffed to its security. I know damned well that if I change jobs, my wife is not going to like it. She can say whatever sounds good, but I know the truth. There's going to be hell to pay if I stop bringing in as much money as I do. I know that *I* could tolerate the stress of the change. I'll just look at it as another challenge to be faced head-on. But I don't know if I want to deal with my marriage being shaken up."

Thus, the marital battles begin. What starts out as an internal struggle between a need for security and a need for a change can end up being a marital struggle. One spouse is "assigned" the role of person pushing for change; the other is assigned the role of voice of reason, warning that the status quo should not be shaken. Caught in this trap, the person going through the career crisis soon begins feeling an urgent need to change *something*. But exactly what needs to be changed becomes unclear: one's career or one's marriage. This is exactly the sort of questioning that filled the life of Jake Landry, the physician whose story we told in Chapter 1.

We sometimes counsel medical couples who are threatening separation because of this relationship trap. Ending the marriage is a tangible, doable act that can bring momentary relief despite its heartbreak and stress. The problem is that in this situation ending the marriage may be fixing a part of life that is *not* broken. Very often the marital tensions that lead to such separations actually are the *effects of*, not the *causes of*, the original drama. Fast-forward six months and these people usually wake up hurt and confused, still burdened with the career crisis that precipitated their problems in the first place.

It's Not All About Psychology. We also have become painfully familiar with a very different flavor of medical marital stress caused by career crisis. In the course of our more than twenty years of practice, a pervasive career insecurity has developed, not only in medicine, but in our general culture. From 1987 to 1994, 85 percent of Fortune 1000 companies laid people off.[8] Physicians, especially, have become distressed, by the ongoing threats to income and career security that come not only from managed care, but also from reports of failed contracts following practice buyouts and practice realignments.[9]

Along the way, we have counseled many hardworking, talented people who were thrown into a career crisis by external, as opposed to psychological, factors.

These were people who became victims of circumstances beyond their control. They lost their jobs for reasons that did not have to do with their job performance. These days, this trauma comes in many shades: cutbacks, scale-downs, economic changes in medicine due to the advent of managed care, layoffs, or simply, "Sorry, you're fired."

For most people, the shock and dismay that come with losing a job are matched only by the self-doubt that follows. We have been sobered by the amount of anxiety such crises have brought to medical couples, and we have been inspired by the ways that many have heroically rallied to support each other.

A career crisis forces reevaluation and redefinition not only of one's lifestyle but also of one's self-concept. This is especially true for those high-powered people who have historically based their self-worth on their ability to perform and maintain control. It is humbling to realize that, no matter how powerful or competent you may be, fate sometimes changes the course of your life.

This type of crisis creates a poignant window of opportunity for a medical couple. Perhaps for the first time, the high-powered spouses undergoing such crisis can learn that they are valued not only for what they *do*, but for who they *are*. For most high-powered people, this is an alien concept. No one is in a more powerful position to deliver this healing message than a partner.

Crisis 6: Lack of Money

Even if your career remains intact, the economic double-cross of modern times is likely to strain your marriage. This is a bitter realization for baby boomers, a generation of educated, ambitious people who assumed that they were doing what was necessary to gain affluence.

Since the mid-1950s, the combination of inflated expectations, inflated cost of living, and the deflated value of the dollar has resulted in more financial stress and disillusionment than most couples planned to face. Many medical couples suffer from measuring themselves with outdated yardsticks of affluence, yardsticks that were created by their medical ancestors. The plight of one of our former clients, physician Allison Mullatte, is a real-life case in point.

"I was scripted to be the golden-haired success story in my family. The first college-educated Mullatte, I was supposed to be the one whose talents were going to help raise my family above our modest, lower-middle-class background.

"When I graduated from high school in 1967, one of the most affluent people in my little southern hometown was Dr. Miller, our general practitioner. He was a very kind and friendly man. I spent summers working in his office, and he seemed to love to talk with me about medicine and what I could expect if I entered his profession. He was nonsexist before the term came in vogue. He also told me that he was living very comfortably on his income of $115,000 per year.

"So I went to medical school, assuming that as long as I made the grades, my future would be assured. Well, my pharmacist-husband and I made $193,000 last year, and we are struggling to stay afloat. Let me rephrase that: We are struggling to adjust to the fact that our version of 'floating' doesn't match our plans about what our life was supposed to be. Once we pay our taxes, mortgage, and living expenses and fund our retirement plan, we basically live from paycheck to paycheck. We do not have enough money for nice vacations or for me to fly home to visit my family as often as I'd like. We can't even afford to send our children to the school of our choice.

"To tell you the truth, I feel sort of like a fraud. My mother and father are obviously proud of me. They love to brag about their 'daughter the doctor' who is seemingly making it 'in the big city, up East.' My dad marvels at the fact that I started out making more than three times what he ever earned. But the truth is that I feel less successful than I look. I'm not talking about wanting a second home and fancy cars; I just want to have enough money to be able to educate my kids and live comfortably.

"I don't really know what to do about this. I sometimes wish that my husband would be more ambitious. He'll never make much money

working for a big pharmacy chain like he does, but his degrees would open some doors in the pharmaceutical industry. If he could manage to up his income, then we'd be more comfortable."

As we travel throughout the country conducting workshops for high-powered people, we often present the story of Allison Mullatte. We do so in order to observe the different reactions of the audience and to help people gain perspective on themselves.

Some people react to Allison's "plight" by questioning: "What is this woman complaining about? Maybe people like the good doctor ought to be reminded of how lucky they are. After all, she does have enough stable income to afford a house, a periodic vacation, and an occasional plane ticket to fly to visit relatives. She is making more money than 90 percent of the people in the world. Let's get some perspective here!"

Others readily empathize with Allison. They agree with the adage that no matter how much income you have, there never seems to be enough money. A modern couple's lifestyle seems to escalate in proportion to their income, and then some. As one of our workshop participants put it: "We are an age of people who live in pursuit of that extra $20,000. Everyone I know moans, 'If only I could get my hands on an extra $20,000, I'd be okay. I'd get in front of this wave of bills that threaten to drown me rather than constantly scrambling to stay afloat.'"

Finally, the story of Allison Mullatte typically helps couples begin to get their own financial dynamic into perspective. Last year, the clients who consulted us reported incomes ranging from less than $15,000 to over $1 million per year. Our experiences suggest that while the extremes of poverty and affluence create certain unique stresses, couples living any-place in between share common relationship risks that revolve around money. No matter how much you earn, it is probably true that money concerns regularly create tension in your relationship. These tensions often have to do with power struggles that get expressed in your dealings with each other about money or with the fact that for many people money gets paired with identity and self-worth.

Money and Marital Struggles. Relationship struggles over money can take many forms. One obvious pattern involves a highly controlling, dominating spouse and a seemingly passive, victimized partner locking horns in a struggle about spending. Here the controller is driven to distraction by the "powerless" partner's relentless refusal to cooperate with the controller's financial plan. In effect, spending serves as the passive partner's power-balancing lever in the marriage. No matter how much the controller argues, preaches, or teaches budgeting and balancing the checkbook, the spender goes on spending according to his or her own plan. The spender's behavior is sending a power-balancing message: "You might be able to outthink me, outtalk me, and outargue me, but I'll be damned if you can control *this* part of our life together."

If you are locked into such a struggle, it is highly likely that other important issues are festering in your relationship. Examining your money struggle probably will lead to further discussion of these underlying issues—this is one reason why so many couples cooperate in remaining locked into an impasse regarding a seemingly simple issue. Even though arguing about the issue may be stressful, doing so may actually be less frightening than dealing with relationship factors that are less quantifiable and more threatening. In this sense, focusing on money matters can be yet another form of the triangulation pattern described in Chapter 5.

Why Don't *You* Get Us Out of This Mess? Less obvious is the plight of many medical couples who have been seduced into living beyond their means and feel ashamed that they cannot afford their lifestyle. The kids are in private school, they live in the "right" section of town, and they worry about "keeping up with the Joneses" (even though they typically deny it). Their private struggle revolves around each of them waiting for the other to find the wisdom and courage to lead them into a more financially comfortable and authentic way of living. The following glimpses into the marriage of Cecile and Martin Peterson show how this can lead to complicated relationship dramas.

Martin: *"I'm getting worn out by this. I feel guilty about the fact that we depend on the generosity of Celie's parents to send our kids to school and pay our taxes. I earn a six-figure income. We ought to be able to live on what I make alone.*

"The problem is the size of our life. As crazy as it sounds, even on my income, we just can't keep living the way we are. We can't have a big house, expensive vacations, the monthly money hemorrhage that comes from eating out three or four times a week and going out on the town every weekend, and still make ends meet.

"I keep saying this, and Cecile keeps agreeing that we are going to have to cut back. Then she gets that disappointed look in her eyes whenever we consider not getting or doing something we want, and I figure, 'Hey, it's just money.' I hate feeling like a wimp and a tightwad. I like feeling like the freewheeling, successful doctor she married."

Cecile: *"If I've told Martin once, I've told him 8,000 times: 'Let's sell this house, buy something more affordable (but nice), and go for comfort rather than for flash.' I've also offered to go back to work in order to help make ends meet.*

"But he *is the one who refuses to consider any of these options. He's*

stuck in his rationalizations: 'It would be a dumb financial move to try to unload the house in the current market.' 'It would cost us more than we would gain if you went to work.' On and on and on.

"I don't like how angry he is about this whole issue. He is being unfair. I know that he blames me for our lifestyle. But the truth is that he's the one who would be embarrassed to have a working wife; it doesn't match his image of himself as Mr. Physician. He's the one who keeps bringing home plans for yet another family-vacation extravaganza. He's the one who keeps coming up with ideas about adding this or that to our house and to our overflowing list of possessions.

"Of course, I get excited about taking nice trips and having nice things. Who wouldn't? But if he would just stop offering them, I would not go searching for them. If he's going to be in charge of the money, then he ought to take charge of the spending, too. He can't have it both ways."

In each of these scenarios, financial strains, resentments over financial power struggles, and plain old fatigue over worrying about money lead to marital tensions. As Frank Farrell, one of our physician friends, is fond of saying, "The American way of life is real simple: When something goes wrong, just keep throwing money at it until it stops wiggling." The problem is that many high-powered couples get stuck in the pattern of attempting solutions to financial problems that just keep creating larger and larger lives, and they never find enough money to stop all of the wiggle.

Crisis 7: Retirement and the Second Half of Marriage

This is such a prevalent and important topic for today's medical marriages that we devote our next chapter to it.

The Risk of Disillusionment

Whether due to the stresses that come with crises or to the confusion that sets in as your relationship grows, disillusionment is a high-risk stage of marriage. Many couples hit disillusionment and then get stuck in a spiraling power struggle, essentially beating their relationship to death.

Declaring Your Loyalty

How can you survive crisis and disillusionment with your romance intact? To begin with, you must renew your loyalty and commitment to your marriage. This can be a scary proposition in the midst of crisis. After all, your very way of reacting to crisis may be reducing your intimacy and fueling your disillusionment. If so, you now have two problems: the crisis *and* your disillusionment. Yet we're *still* preaching that you need to toss your hat resolutely into the ring of the marriage.

Our reason for this is simple. Crisis forces you to face a crucial question: What and whom are you going to choose to value as you restructure your life on the all-important *next* level?

How *you* choose to react will shape the teamwork that evolves in your marriage, and this teamwork will determine the quality of your relationship. Put another way: Whether your marriage becomes a major source of distress or a major source of comfort during disillusionment will depend largely on *you*, not on what has happened to *you* and not on your mate.

Life crises—including those in your marriage—create opportunities for heroism in relationships, opportunities to attain new levels of trust and intimacy, even though the relationship *itself* may seem like your major stress. But this will happen only *if* you are willing to take responsibility for yourselves and be there for each other—lovingly.

What does this involve? How can you move beyond your struggles and your growing fear that the problem in your life *is* your marriage?

References

1. Kiecolt-Glaser JK, Glaser R, Cacioppo JT, et al. Marital conflict in older adults: endocrinological and immunological correlates. *Psychosom Med.* 1997;59:339-349.
2. Gottman J, Silver N. *The Seven Principles for Making Marriage Work.* New York, NY: Cron Pub; 1999.
3. McCue J. Doctors and stress: is there really a problem? *Hosp Pract.* 1986;21:7-16.
4. Robinson DO. The medical-student spouse syndrome: grief reactions to the clinical years. *Am J Psychiatry.* 1978;135:972-974.
5. Myers M. *Doctors' Marriages: A Look at the Problems and Their Solutions.* New York, NY: Plenum Publishing; 1988.
6. Gonzalez ML. *Medical Professional Liability Trends, 1985-1997.* Chicago, Ill: American Medical Association Center for Health Policy Research; 1999.
7. Reading EG. The malpractice stress syndrome. *N Engl J Med.* 1986;83:289-290.
8. Senator Thomas A. Daschle. *Congressional Record.* April 2, 1993. Cited by: Reinhold BB. *Toxic Work.* New York, NY: Dutton; 1996.
9. Zewick P. Some doctors quit hospital deals: transfer of primary-care practices wasn't magic pill they expected. *Winston-Salem Journal.* October 18, 1999:1.

Chapter 7

Dancing in the Empty Nest

*It takes guts to stay married . . . . There will be many
crises between the wedding day and the golden
anniversary, and the people who make it are heroes.*

—Howard Whiteman,
Philadelphia Sunday Bulletin; January 15, 1967

August 1999 was a momentous month for us. We received word from the
AMA of their interest in purchasing the rights to *The Medical Marriage,*
we packed our younger daughter off to college, and Mary celebrated her
fiftieth birthday. Just as the "I do" and "It's a girl!" proclamations had
abruptly changed our lives, we once again found ourselves in totally new
territory: a big, empty nest filled with new opportunities.

The second half of marriage is an interesting paradox. By this stage,
you've become exquisitely familiar with your relationship dances. You've
grown accustomed to the roles you've assumed and assigned to each other
as you've moved through the decades. Your own shorthand nuances have
streamlined your ways of communicating with each other. After a couple
of decades of being together, the sequences and patterns of your intimacy,
conflict, and daily living have taken on a certain predictability. You've
heard each other's stories. You can finish each other's sentences. You are
deeply familiar to each other.

But the second half is also a new beginning, a time to stretch from
the familiar and to embrace new opportunities. This necessitates learning
new ways of perceiving each other and of interacting. It also requires that
you bear through your awkwardness as you learn new steps in old dances.

As we enter the new millennium, record numbers of couples are facing the challenge of adapting to their empty nest. As of 1999, 35 million Americans were sixty-five or over, and 4 million were over age eighty-five. By the year 2030, both of these figures are expected to double. By 2040, nearly a quarter of the American population will be sixty-five and older.[1]

The physician population is no exception. According to the American Medical Association, in the United States alone, there are approximately 756,710 practicing physicians. Of these, approximately 17 percent were age sixty-five or older in 1997. The total number of physicians sixty-five and over tripled from 38,146 in 1970 to 129,692 in 1997. In addition, 14 percent of active physicians today are fifty-five to sixty-five years of age, and 409,468 are beyond forty-five years of age.[2]

Similar statistics apply to physicians worldwide. For example, in Canada, 10.7 percent of "active" physicians in 1996 were sixty-five years or older, while 15.9 percent ranged in age from fifty-five to sixty-four.[3] The mean age of Canadian physicians who retired in 1995 and 1996 was sixty-eight.

We present these statistics simply to make this point: Record numbers of medical families are currently or imminently facing the dual challenges of adjusting to midlife family issues and retirement. In both our clinical practice and consulting, we frequently glimpse the issues and the opportunities that face such couples.

Austin and Jarrod

Austin, wife of surgeon, Jarrod: *"I have to admit, all this talk of taking early retirement scares me. The truth is that I don't know how we will handle it if he retires. What will he do with himself? He's such a stimulation-seeker, I'm afraid that he'll expect me to just up and travel all over creation with him, whether I want to or not—and I don't want to! I like my life just like it is. Our daughter just had our first grandchild, and I love being a hands-on grandma. Plus, I worry about how we will handle Jarrod being home all the time. He's used to being in charge at his office, and, God knows, he's in charge in the OR. But this house is my territory.*

"I sort of think it might be better for him to keep working a while longer. Maybe cut back some, but keep doing surgery."

Jarrod, surgeon: *"I've been working hard since I was a kid. More and more, I find myself thinking about hanging it up, and seeing what the other half lives like. I know that Austin is nervous about this. So am I; I've never not worked. But I'm tired and frustrated, and I want a change.*

"Austin keeps encouraging me to slow down, and not stop. That's easier said than done. No one in our practice has ever 'slowed down.' The model of practice has been 'work till you drop.' Literally, that's what

the founding surgeons did in our group: Each of them worked until they died. Not only do I not know how to be a half-speed surgeon; no one in my profession seems to know how to help a surgeon change pace."

Caroline and Luke

Caroline, spouse of a physician: *"Let me tell you what I think about the empty nest: I love it! I hadn't realized how much my worrying about day-to-day parenting detracted from my putting energy into making our marriage better. Since our kids left home, things have just gotten better and better for Luke and me."*

Luke, physician: *"I agree. Caroline and I have always had a strong marriage, but now, we're back to having a fun marriage. And I guarantee you, things will get another notch better when I retire in two years. I can't wait. I've loved practicing medicine; but I also love a lot of stuff that I just haven't had the time or energy to do."*

Joseph and Stephanie

Stephanie, nurse: *"Everyone said this stage of life would be over before we knew it, so enjoy it while it lasts. They were right on. Now, that they're over, I look around at our big, empty house, and wonder where all those years went.*

"But the surprise is how differently Joseph and I are reacting to this empty nest. Our youngest son just got married. What a bittersweet moment that was for us. I feel so ready to celebrate our life and our kids' being adults. I feel ready to slow down and enjoy our success—we raised a great family, and we've each had a wonderful medical career. But Joseph looked so sad all through our son's wedding. He has difficulty talking about his feelings, but I know that he's not quite ready for this stage of life."

Joseph, physician: *"As I sat in that church, watching our youngest son get married, the litany of questions that have been filling my head for a year continued. I'm questioning every major choice I made in my life and the choices I'm considering making. 'What would life have been like if I hadn't become a physician?' 'Why do I spend so much time working?' 'Is it really time for me to retire, or am I just going along with Stephanie's momentum?'"*

"She seems to be so much more actualized about all of this than I am. She obviously feels completed. She's had enough hands-on parenting and nursing, and now she's ready to chart some new territory. I'm not sure that I've had enough hands-on anything. Seems like I've spent the past 30 years in my head. Now, just when I'm ready to join my family, they're spinning out into worlds of their own. Just when I've supposedly earned the right to slow down and smell the roses, I'm not sure which roses I want to smell."

Letting Go as They Grow

Many couples are shocked into noticing their marital issues only when they face the midlife transition, signaled either by their children's entry into late adolescence and early adulthood or their own retirement. These passages in individual development correspond to stages of marriage that often invoke feelings that are hard to identify and even harder to work through.

Typical are feelings of sadness or, at minimum, nostalgia about what is ending—the need to maintain a nest for the family. These feelings may be coupled with anxiety and awkwardness about what is to come, both professionally and personally. By this stage of life, most medical couples are so accustomed to organizing themselves around their roles as parents and members of the medical profession that those roles have come to define and organize the marriage. The challenge in the second half is to create new meaning—as individuals and as a couple. Many couples fail to clear this hurdle. The National Center of Health Statistics reported that, while the overall divorce rate in the United States declined from 1981 to 1991, divorce among couples married thirty years or more showed a sharp increase. The overall divorce rate decreased 1.4 percent during that decade, while divorce in the thirty-year plus marriages increased 16 percent.[4]

In this chapter, we will discuss several normative crises faced by aging medical couples and offer advice about how to make the second half the best part of a medical marriage.

You Mean I'm Never Going to Be President?

No matter how much we do, how much we achieve, or how happy we are with our lives, part of our journey through adulthood involves coming to grips with the fact that our lives might have gone quite differently. For some, this means grieving over lost dreams.

For others, crisis comes in the form of realizing that even though a major quest has come to fruition ("I am the president!"), life would have been quite different and enjoyable in other ways if different choices had been made. Each year in our practice we hear numerous president types (doctors, lawyers, CEOs, one and all) who admit, "I sometimes wish that I had gone for a simpler life, like my brother [or neighbor]. He seems to be so calm and contented. He goes to work, comes home, and enjoys filling in the leftover time in his life with interesting hobbies and relationships. I like what I'm doing, but this career has filled my life. There just hasn't been room for other things that I know I would have enjoyed just as much, maybe more."

No matter what our station in life, each of us spends at least some energy pondering the goals we did not reach, considering roads we did not travel, and fantasizing about relationships we did not pursue. This does not mean that we are filled with regret. It simply means that we are more limited in time than in our capacity to be and do all that we potentially could.

A variation of this theme is questioning the choices that shape marriage and family. The range of questions are endless. To name but a few that we frequently hear from our clients:

- "I wonder what it might have been like if we had become parents."
- "I sometimes wish we'd had more children."
- "I wonder what life would have been like if we'd had fewer children."
- "I wish we had not decided to have an abortion."
- "I wish I had parented differently."
- "I wish you had parented differently."
- "I wish we had decided to get sober sooner than we did."
- "Life would have been so different for us if we had lived someplace else."
- "What would our life be like if we had different kinds of careers?"
- "I sometimes question how we have dealt with religion in our lives."
- "If only we had managed our money differently."

Every couple makes some choices—either individually or collectively—that they regret. The guilt, shaming, blaming, and recrimination that often come with questioning such choices can create a marital crisis. The historical event can't be erased, the consequences often cannot be undone, and the wounded person or persons face a fundamental choice: forgive and go on, or hold on to anger and resentment and run the risk of ruining the here-and-now relationship by wallowing in disillusionment.

Midlife Questioning and Midlife Crisis

Conservatively estimated, one third of the physician-clients we see are experiencing a self- or partner-diagnosed "midlife crisis." In truth, they are often not as much in crisis as they are questioning the fit between the way they are living their life and the way they would like to live, and their judgment is being questioned by those around them. It seems to us that the so-called midlife crisis syndrome typically develops as follows:

- In step 1, someone who is, according to his or her spouse, "definitely old enough to know better" begins to figure out what he or she really thinks, needs, feels, or wants.
- Step 2 begins when this person finally finds the courage to express this newly discovered information.
- Step 3 quickly follows. Everyone who has anything to do with this

newly enlightened person immediately goes into crisis, especially anyone who will have to change if this person begins acting on this new awareness.

• Step 4 usually comes sooner than later. The person doing the questioning is dragged into counseling by a confused and frightened spouse, and the counselor is charged with the responsibility of convincing this questioning person to "go back to behaving in ways he or she used to behave."

The stereotypical "midlife crisis"—a balding man who tries to run from middle age by changing his body, his acquaintances, and his career—actually occurs in less than 10 percent of the middle-aged population. In the stereotypical "midlife crisis," this man begins to chase younger women, justifying his actions by blaming his "boring spouse." Amid this self-centered and irresponsible frenzy, he seems intent on abdicating all of his marital and family responsibilities.

We have counseled thousands of middle-aged men and women, some of whom have pursued relationships with people younger than themselves. However, few of these individuals have even come close to abdicating their personal or professional responsibilities. Most often, they are thoughtful people who are grappling with their healthy need to develop more authenticity in their lives. They are struggling to find a better fit between what they are doing with their precious life's energies and what they want and need to do in order to be true to themselves and responsible to the commitments that define their lives.

Middle age is a rich, complex, powerful time of life—for most, a time of bravery, capability, and fatigue. When—not if—midlife questioning begins, it is imperative that a couple commit themselves to developing whatever skills are required to negotiate a successful resolution of the dilemmas.

Several factors may converge to add to a rather rude midlife awakening in any contemporary medical couple:

• The status and prestige that you expected from this profession may materialize only partly, if at all.
• The long-awaited rejoining after prolonged periods of intense career demands may never fully materialize. The anticipated midcareer slowdown never arrives.
• You will probably not prove to be exceptions to any of the typical struggles that characterize marriage and family life.

These same statements could apply to couples whose lives revolve around many professions. But we believe that, due to the unique demands of the medical profession and to the aforementioned personality-based tendencies of physicians and their loved ones, medical couples are at risk of settling into a particular pattern of marital disillusionment that magnifies midlife questioning. This medical-marriage disillusionment stage is signaled by seven characteristics.[5]

1. Intimacy gradually erodes.
2. Open expression of emotions to each other stops.
3. Communication gets stilted as discussion of touchy or troubling issues is avoided.
4. Sexual relations dwindle and become less enjoyable.
5. You develop separate lives: your interests and involvements diverge to the point that you have little in common.
6. You begin to "cooperate" in mutual withdrawal. The typical pursuer gives up; as a couple, you settle into a pattern of emotional distance.
7. The stress of your lifestyle becomes the glue that holds you together. As a result, both of you develop a vested interest in continuing the stress; if it disappears, so may your marriage.

Of course, it doesn't have to be this way. Healthy medical couples resolve midlife questioning by shifting the way they organize their time as well as their perceptions of each other. More about this later.

When Important People Leave Your Family

Your marriage will be at risk when people enter or leave the family. A new arrival is usually counterbalanced by the joy of what is gained: the new baby, in-law, or friends who become like family. But when people depart, a hole is left that automatically fills with longing for the lost loved one and with anxiety about the resulting awkwardness in family relationships that have to be renegotiated. This can be a confusing time as everyone scrambles to adjust to the change.

Even Small Steps Can Hurt. For some families, these periods of confusion come in small doses all along the way.

One of our female clients recently showed up for her appointment in tears. "What's wrong?" I asked.

"I'm just sad about my daughter growing up so fast. I'm not ready for this. I love being a mom. I don't want it to end."

I was puzzled by her tears. "Wait a minute. Isn't your daughter only six years old?"

"Yes." (More tears) "But she learned to ride a two-wheel bicycle yesterday, and it broke my heart. I saw her riding down that sidewalk, and I knew that it wouldn't be long before she'll be driving away from me forever."

In addition to simply loving her daughter and thriving in her role as a mother, this woman also feared the emptiness that she felt in her marriage. Her daughter's growth reminded her that she and her husband had bridges to build in order to reconnect with each other. Thankfully, these people are already paying attention to this, even at this early stage of family life.

Even if you are joyous about your children growing more independent, launching them from your family and into their own worlds can be stressful. For one thing, children often batter the nest as they get ready to fly, separating—at least emotionally—by stirring conflict within the family. They bolster their courage by practicing living "alone" while residing under the same roof as their parents.

Today, record numbers of couples face the challenge of dealing with the boomerang generation phenomenon. Speaking of her two grown children, one of our patients put it this way: "We educated them, launched them, married them, and they boomeranged back and lived in our basement and on our payroll until they were forty-two!" In the 1990s, one in five middle-aged parents had an adult child still living in the nest. In fact, more than one third of unmarried American men between ages of twenty-five and thirty-four still live at home.[6]

And if That's Not Bad Enough, Try This. For many couples, the challenges that come when children leave home (or boomerang back!) are compounded by the stresses that come from living in the "sandwich" generation. Just as your children are launching, your own aging parents are likely to need increased attention. It has been estimated that by the year 2020, the typical family will consist of at least four generations and that by 2040 nearly a quarter of the American population will be sixty-five and older.[7] By then, middle-generation women may spend more years with parents over sixty-five than with children under eighteen, and a high percentage of these aging adults will need hands-on and financial aid from their middle-aged children as they face rising health care and living costs and increased financial vulnerability. In 1999, one in twenty middle-aged parents had a parent living with them.[7]

Even if you manage to escape the pressures of providing physical care for your aging parents, you are likely to have to deal with the psychological pressures that come when they need increased connection with you. As old age approaches, even the most uninvolved parent gravitates toward a connection with family or with his or her history as a way of making amends or simply out of loneliness, fear, or need.

This can create tremendous conflict for middle-aged people who have settled into a comfortable closeness or distance from their aged parents.

Moving Closer to Aging Parents

Moving closer to parents who have been hurtful may feel artificial and distressing. In some instances, like the case of Edie that opened Chapter 6 and continues below, reconnecting with a parent is fraught with fear of undoing the progress that has been made at the expense (and pain) of giving up hope of ever having a loving parental relationship.

Three years after her divorce from Simon, Edie returned to us for help. She and her two brothers had been reared in a family that revolved around the chaos caused by her father's alcoholism. He had verbally and sexually abused Edie, and she was terrified of him and resentful of her mother for not protecting her. Even as an adult, she had suffered the effects of this upbringing. Before her ill-fated marriage to Simon, Edie went through periods of promiscuity, drug abuse, and compulsive spending.

Following her divorce from Simon, Edie had a backslide. Eventually, she entered an impaired-physicians program for treatment of her addictions to alcohol and amphetamines. Following her inpatient treatment, she courageously confronted herself during a four-year course of therapy. She remained sober, reexamined her codependent tendencies in close relationships, and, for the first time in her life, began taking care of herself.

But her hard-earned sense of well-being was threatened when her mother made plans to move to a suburb of the city in which Edie lived. The mother wanted to spend her last years near her daughter. Edie's reaction was understandable:

"It took me firty-five years to learn what I wish my parents had taught me: I am a loving and lovable person. I finally believe this about myself.

"That's why this is so hard. The fact that I do not want my mother to live closer to me violates my understanding of myself as a loving person. Plus, there's the lesson that you drilled home to me in our first round of therapy: 'You won't be healthy unless and until you find the guts it takes to create nurturing territory and to stay out of toxic territory. This starts with paying attention to your relationships.'

"I spent so much of my life 'looking for love in all the wrong places,' as the song says. I spent so much time confused about which relationships to stay in, which to pursue, and which to end. But no more. For the first time, my life is filled with people who make me feel good. I know that this is important to my survival.

"What am I supposed to do about the fact that I do not feel good—I don't even feel safe—when I am around my mother for any length of time? Since she mentioned moving here, I have been waking up with anxiety attacks. Maybe I need to try to come to some new level of peace with her. I don't know. I just know that I don't feel good about her being any major part of my life.

"But something else is definitely true: She is just an old lady who is scared, and I no longer need for her to protect me from my father. The

man is dead, for heaven's sake! Now I'm the powerful one. I'm a middle-aged woman; I'm a successful physician; and I know how to take care of myself.

"I know all of that, but I don't know what to do about this dilemma."

There were no ready-made answers to Edie's quandary. She struggled with this dilemma throughout the last three years of her mother's life. She was able to endure—but never enjoy—her mother's presence. Her friends and various support systems helped her remain healthy as she faced this last drama with her mother.

Fortunately, most people don't have as much pain in their parental relationships as Edie. But even when we have caring relationships with our aging parents, trying to find time and space in our busy lives for increased connection with them can be a problem. When we are already trying to do more than is humanly possible, incorporating the care of an aging parent can create stress overload for individuals and families.

Moving Away From Aging Parents

Letting go of our parents as they grow old, experience illness, or approach death is stressful, if not heartbreaking. Few things change the meaning of life more abruptly than the death of a parent. At such times, we are reminded that this is no dress rehearsal; this is the only life we get. We also are faced with the anxiety, awkwardness, and freedom that come from claiming our positions as the front-runners in our families.

As you grieve the actual or anticipated loss of a loved one, you begin to examine more closely the relationships that remain in your life. Hopefully, what we feel, see, and hear in return will lead to renewed appreciation for the people who remain in our lives—and also to finding the courage to do what family therapist Terry Hargrave calls "finishing well."[8] Finishing well means finding the courage to deal directly with each other about whatever transgenerational issues need to be acknowledged, if not resolved, as the last days of a family member's life approach.

The Second Half of Medical Marriage

You know your marriage is in the second half when . . .

- You have teenagers who will soon leave the nest.
- Your own parents are aging
- You were recently invited to your twenty-fifth high school reunion.
- You exercise more and burn fewer calories doing it.
- You just received an invitation to join AARP.
- By the time you get your spouse's attention, you've forgotten what you were going to say.[9]

In their wonderful book, *The Second Half of Marriage: Facing the Eight Challenges of Every Long-Term Marriage*, David and Claudia Arp[9] remind us that advancing years bring couples many opportunities. These include the opportunities to get reacquainted; to rejuvenate your friendship and your sexual relationship; to expand your personal boundaries; to reconcile your differences; and to come to peace with aging parents and negotiate new relationships with your grown children.

Contrary to popular mythology, recent research clearly shows that middle age is the prime of life. In its 1999 report on a ten-year study of 2,727 Americans, ages twenty-five to seventy-four, the MacArthur Foundation Research Network on Successful Midlife Development found that between the ages of thirty-five and sixty-five, and in particular between forty and sixty, people report increased feelings of well-being, optimism, happiness, and youthful outlook.[10] Most middle-aged people say they feel better about their lives than they did ten years before.

And an encouraging addendum to the aforementioned, sobering statistic about the 1981-to-1991 rise in divorce rates among aging couples: A majority of the middle-aged Americans in the MacArthur survey reported that their marriages or relationships were stable and relatively happy. In fact, 72 percent of the spouses in the MacArthur Foundation study described their marriages as being "excellent" or "very good," and 90 percent voiced confidence that their marriages would last. But this stage of marriage is not without its challenges.

Development Never Stops

Psychologist Erik Erikson was the first to conceptualize how psychological development progresses through all the stages of the life cycle. Subsequent researchers have shown that this concept applies not only to our individual, emotional development, but also to our cognitive and family functioning.

For both genders, midlife is a time when wisdom blossoms. Contrary to popular mythology that we "lose IQ points" as we age, several mental functions actually *improve* with age.[11] These include the ability to problem-solve with wisdom borne from decades' of experience, the ability to fluidly think through problems, and the ability to draw from a wide vocabulary when describing our experiences.

During midlife, we are also compelled to move beyond whatever role has heretofore predominated in our life and begin to give expression to some heretofore underexpressed part of our self. Often, this creates interesting twists in a family's teamwork. How many of you have heard or said something like the following: "John, you *never* treated our kids like you treat those grandkids—spoiling them, tolerating their rambunctious behavior. Where was all that tenderness when our kids were babies?" Or:

"I'll tell you what: As she's gotten older, mom sure has gotten feisty! She speaks her mind, no matter who's listening. She never used to be like that."

These changes are due to what's called the midlife crossover. It goes like this: As they age, women tend to move from being relationship focused to being more assertive, expressive, or ambitious. Men, on the other hand, who typically have been out in the world, often express an increased need for connection and greater intimacy at this time of life. This process is depicted below.

The Midlife Crossover[12]

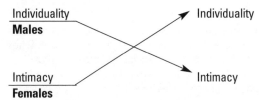

For many women, midlife is a time of stretching their focus, either outside of the home for the first time, further into already-established careers, or back to the nest they have absented for too much of their early adulthood. For others, this is simply a time of first discovering and then expressing their own voice: what they really think, feel, need, or want.

While midlife is a woman's time to fly, this doesn't mean she becomes the president of IBM or goes to law school at age seventy, although it may mean that. It means she embraces the power she has to make choices in her life, based on the wisdom she has gained about herself and the world. When women come to trust their wisdom and begin to tell the truth about what they think, feel, want, and need in their lives, the significant others in their lives must listen.[13]

The wisdom of middle age compels men to counterbalance the excessive work focus that fills their early adulthood with more nurturing, playful experiences. Our clinical experiences suggest that aging doctors face challenges similar to those encountered by aging executives. Ron Halpern, author of *Quiet Desperation*, reported on a nationwide survey of 4,000 male executives, managers, physicians, lawyers, and accountants between the ages of twenty-seven and seventy-eight.[14] Fifty percent of the senior professionals polled regretted spending so many hours at their jobs; 68 percent were quite happy with professional life, but lamented how their family life had suffered in deference to their careers. Fully 58 percent felt they had wasted years striving for and achieving success that they now found to be "empty and meaningless." The defining characteristics of the 23 percent of older, "satisfied and happy" executives in the Halpern study constitute advice worthy of heeding by professionals of any age.

The satisfied and happy senior professionals were committed to relearning how to have fun at work; they valued personal growth, intimate friendships, and family relationships; and they had learned to move beyond their lifelong pursuits of status, fame, and financial success.

For most middle-aged male physicians, the world makes this especially difficult to do. The extreme work demands that come with being a physician, coupled with societal expectations that physicians be all things to all people, compound the dilemma faced by all males in our culture: balancing achievement striving with appropriate self-care.

Unfortunately, in the ways they treat each other, men tend to compound their own struggles. Psychiatrist Frank Pittman described this process:

> Masculinity is a group activity. As a guy develops and practices his masculinity, he is critiqued by an invisible male chorus of all the other guys, who hiss or cheer as he attempts to approximate the masculine ideal, who push him to sacrifice more and more of his humanity, who ridicule him when he holds back. This chorus is made up of comrades and rivals, his buddies and bosses, his male ancestors and his male cultural heroes—and, above all, his father.[15]

For many men, an effect of this brutal chorus is failure to develop appropriate self-nurturing skills. Because they lack appropriate societal, professional, or peer support to incorporate more nurturing into their lives, many male physicians become excessively dependent on their mates to fill this need. The midlife crossover phenomenon may deeply threaten such a man, leaving him to feel unloved and angry. An aging couple must learn to understand and accept that the midlife crossover indicates a healthy and natural developmental blossoming; it's about growth, not dependency or abandonment.

The process of a couple stretching to accommodate each other's growth during this second stage is a beautiful thing to observe. But even the most harmonious of medical couples will be challenged as retirement from the "great mistress—medicine" approaches.

Retirement

Many physicians cannot imagine life without medicine. For them, medicine is a priesthood; it's a lifetime thing.[16] But statistics show that, with rare exception, the majority of physicians hang up their stethoscopes approximately forty years after getting their medical degree—some time between their late sixties and early seventies.

These days, many younger doctors look forward to retiring at an even earlier age. For example, management consultants in Canada have reported that, in growing numbers, physicians as young as in their early thirties are attending retirement workshops.[16]

How Can You Slow Down on the Fast Track?

Retirement can be a daunting endeavor for medical families. Too often, physicians have observed their patients enduring the painful scenario depicted by physician Robert Moser: "You know the story. After 6 months he was bored unto despair, and at 12 months was unrelentingly depressed. Within 2 years he was dead."[17]

The case vignette of Jarrod that opened this chapter points out another hurdle encountered by aging physicians: the relative lack of precedents and organizational policies that allow mature physicians to gradually modify their work schedules as they approach retirement. We believe that filling this void is one of the most important challenges faced by medicine and medical families today. Too often, discussion of work/family issues narrowly focuses on the concerns of younger medical families. New models that allow young and older medical families to honor each other's needs are needed.

Developing ways for physicians to slow down and to retire, both with dignity and with the support of their colleagues, requires more than creative financial and work-flow formularies; it also requires an altering of egos that have long been bolstered by the suffering contest that too often is the practice of medicine. One hurdle here is the relative dearth in medicine of precedents for senior partners passing the baton of overwork to the upcoming generation. Unlike many other professions, such as law, it is rare for a medical group to smoothly operate when senior physicians try to maintain high levels of income while also slowing down their professional productivity.

This problem is compounded when an aging physician resists accepting any diminishment in power, income, or prestige commensurate with his or her withdrawal from the front-line delivery of clinical, research, or administrative services. Such resistance leads some physicians to deny their need to retire, a situation that can lead to results that are both embarrassing and risky. If an organization fails to develop realistic, fair ways of assessing an aging physician's capabilities to continue practicing, they may leave themselves vulnerable to having an aging, impaired physician continuing to practice without constraints.

On the other hand, some physicians argue that in medicine, as in other professions, a mandatory retirement age unnecessarily prohibits many wise medical elders from continuing to contribute to their profession and to their communities. Consultants in this field generally agree that many of the dilemmas faced by aging physicians could be circumvented by institutional support of physician retreading. By becoming involved in aspects of medical care, administration, research, or teaching that are less physically demanding and more commensurate with their careerwide accumulation of skills and knowledge, many physicians could extend their years of professional productivity and enjoyment.

Start Early

No definitive research has yet been published regarding the issues faced by retiring physicians. A 1999 literature search through *Index Medicus* indicated that most of the published studies on this subject are descriptive surveys that questioned physicians who had reached the mandatory age for retirement regarding their plans for leaving practice, reasons for retiring, and whether they will continue to engage in medical activity.[18] This literature generally suggests that physicians who seek earlier retirement report a number of reasons for doing so, including concerns related to how malpractice is governed, health-care reform, the high cost of practice, frustration about third-party reimbursement, and diminishing satisfaction with work.

In addition, these publications caution that, due to the tendency to build one's entire identity around being a doctor, retirement is likely to be especially difficult for physicians.[19,20] When patients' needs no longer rule the day, physicians must face the challenge of discovering new facets of themselves.

Testimonials from retired physicians who claim to be happy and thriving suggest a number of guidelines for medical couples of all ages:

- Retire as part of a self-directed plan that involves retiring in order to get to do other things deemed to be desirable.
- Start early in your career to ensure that you will have adequate financial resources upon retiring.
- Retire while you still have at least the perception of good health.
- Learn to enjoy a range of activities outside of medicine.
- Without question, recognize that the decision to retire is a marital/family issue, not an individual issue.

In an eloquently written article published in the *Annals of Internal Medicine*, physician Robert Moser recommends that you begin early to think of retirement as your final career. "It is a career, and it will require every bit as much scheming and planning as any of your other careers . . . Retirement provides the opportunity to explore the vast, wonderful universe that the arduous pursuit of medicine virtually precluded."[17]

Dr. Moser also cautions that the most sensitive aspect of successful retirement is frequently overlooked: marital intimacy.

Creating a New Normal

Both retirement and the second half of marriage are opportunities to take forward the best aspects of your past and merge them with new ways of managing yourselves and interacting with each other to create a friendship-based relationship. It is on this basis that mature romance can blossom. To do so, though, certain pitfalls have to be avoided.

Typically, couples move from being child-focused and career-focused during their first half to becoming activity-focused in their second half. Others settle into lethargy: They build up anticipation that after the kids are grown or the career dramas calm, there will be opportunity to do some of those things they've put off, only to find themselves "double-crossed" by some combination of lost health, diminished physical stamina, lessened sexual energy, dwindled social contacts, and eroded intimacy. Faced with these hurdles, many couples settle into living semi-miserably ever after. The alternative is worth fighting for.

The Arps caution that, if your life goes like most peoples', the second half of your marriage will last as long or longer than the first half.[9] This is an opportunity to build a partner-focused marriage; one that revolves around a closer friendship, new goals, new life experiences, new interests and hobbies, and, perhaps, a new profession. This is also a time to polish your influence on your adult children and grandchildren.

Second-half marital growth depends on your being willing to develop new ways of relating to each other. In our experience, this starts with taking stock of what you need to forgive and change, and typically continues with subtle changes in the following areas:

- How you schedule your time
- How you divide responsibilities
- How you face the challenges of aging healthily
- What you do about your sex life and your nonsexual physical affection.

Step 1: Take Stock. Our own work with medical couples in their mid-forties and older reminds us of a concept philosophers call natural piety: We must learn to look backward with pride in order to find peace, contentment and hope for the future.

This is a time to take stock of yourself and your marriage, and to put to rest some of your age-old struggles. It's a time to forgive yourself and your partner, and to embrace the good fruits of your labors thus far. You can begin to do so by answering the following series of questions recommended by the Arps[9]:

- What have been our marriage liabilities? *Examples:* We live in chronic time pressure. We tend to be lazy about romance. We habitually overspend. We're overinvolved with extended family or our own kids.
- What are the best aspects of our marriage? *Examples:* We have learned to forgive each other, despite the issues we struggle with. We have a strong friendship. Our passion is still alive. We have raised three wonderful children.
- When we finish the race, what do we want our marriage to look like?

- Starting now, what changes can we make that will take us at least a few steps toward being the sort of couple we want to be?

Step 2: Develop New Habits to Spend Time Together. The task here is to gradually create opportunities to regularly spend small chunks of enjoyable time together, just as you did early in your courtship. There's a lesson to learn here from retired couples who report high levels of happiness. They tend to describe how their relationship shifted to more "we-ness" upon entry into retirement. This we-ness may take many forms, each having the common denominator of the couple spending more time together.

For many, this is a time to find the courage it takes to bear through the awkwardness that comes with spending more time together. For most, this requires learning how to set limits on those things that take you out of your relationship. This typically means making small changes that make more frequent contact possible. The experience of Bobby was a case in point.

It's amazing to me what a difference this little change has made in my home life. For more than twenty years, I had the same pattern: I scheduled my last office appointment at 4:45 each day, then scrambled to get my dictation done and rounds at the hospital, all the while rushing to get home sometime between 7:00 and 8:00 PM. Even if I made it home by 7:30, inevitably I was exhausted. I now see how my marriage suffered from my chronic fatigue.

I regret that it took a crisis to get my attention, but I'm happy about the results. When my wife threatened to leave me, I decided to take more control of my time. The realities of having two kids in college, uncertain income, and rising overhead forced me to give up my fantasy/plan of working like a Trojan 'just a few more years,' then retiring young. Those 'few more years' seemed to never come to completion. That's what my wife got tired of telling me. If she said it once, she said it one thousand times: 'If we are going to have a marriage, you need to more regularly be present, complete with at least a modicum of energy and enthusiasm.'

When she agreed to give me one more chance, I got serious about protecting my time. It was hard to do, but I did it. And the amazing thing is how little it took to improve things. I insisted on stopping my office schedule at 4:00 each afternoon. That gave me time to finish my day in a reasonable state of calm and show up at home in a better mood.

Of course, it doesn't always work out. Our evenings aren't always great. Our issues are still our issues. But we spend at least twenty or thirty minutes most evenings talking—with me awake and paying attention. It's amazing what an overall difference this simple change has made.

It would be remiss of us to imply that learning to spend more time together is an easy task. Remember that you have spent the bulk of your marriage thus far out of each other's presence. This will take some getting used to!

Bearing your differences in mind, start now experimenting with various ways to spend time together. This is a learned process. The following list points out but a few examples. Try some; you'll learn to like it!

- Increase how frequently you team up to do even small chores, like making the bed or doing grocery shopping.
- Share a hobby or learn something about your partner's hobby and discuss what you've learned.
- Renew your joint participation in spiritual rituals.
- Create more frequent times to have brief, casual chats.
- Travel together more frequently.
- Share time together with your children or grandchildren.

Step 3: Redistribute Responsibilities. The second half is a time to at least notice, and possibly adjust, the balance of the various roles that each of you play. Again, the words of retired physician, Robert Moser: "I wish I could say we divided the chores. We do not. My wife does much more than I. Yet I am beginning to see what needs to be done. A small point perhaps, but it has to do with fairness and keeping the peace."[17]

Step 4: Commit Yourselves to Helping Each Other Do What Is Possible to Age Well. In a thought-provoking review of gerontology research, John Rowe and Robert Kahn emphasized that, when considering the many factors we typically associate with aging (such as diminished memory and intellectual capability, increased illness, substance abuse, and depression), "Age itself is not a sufficient explanatory variable."[21] Rather, the choices we make starting in midlife chart the course that our aging will take. These and other gerontology researchers have shed light on guidelines for aging well to which couples of all ages should pay attention.

First, remember that "If you don't use it, you'll lose it." This quote is from the famed sex researchers William Masters and Virginia Johnson. Their admonition applies not only to one's sex life, but also to such vital functions as memory, intelligence, and physical flexibility.

The sad fact is that, upon retirement, many people stop exercising their minds and bodies, and many couples sabotage each other's efforts to grow. Thriving couples, on the other hand, tend to have partners who not only encourage but also participate with their forays into new territory. *As a couple*, they explore new interests and stay active. Particularly beyond age seventy-five, the benefits of exercising one's memory through such pastimes as playing bridge, reading, or memorizing for the sake of "keeping in practice" has been shown to help maintain intellectual flexibility.

Perhaps even sadder is the fact that so many couples participate in lifestyles that actively work against aging well. The odds of aging well increase tremendously if you help each other attend to the basics: Get regular exercise, including aerobic, flexibility, and weight-bearing exercises; maintain healthy eating habits; keep alcohol use to a minimum; and, by all means, don't smoke.

This might seem like self-evident advice. But consider these sobering facts. In the aforementioned MacArthur Foundation study of midlife, seven of ten respondents were overweight, and only 23 percent stated that they worked hard to stay healthy. Furthermore, the majority of smokers did not believe they have a higher-than-average risk of developing cancer or heart disease. This denial despite the indisputable medical research that has demonstrated the detrimental effects of poor fitness and health habits! The MacArthur Foundation data lend further support to the observation that, while most Americans enjoy remarkably good health from thirty-five to sixty-five, poor physical fitness and self-destructive habits create a time bomb that threatens an entire generation of aging Americans with increased heart and lung diseases.

In her succinct summary of the practical implications of the best research available on aging well, Betty Friedan offers ten keys to sustaining a vital life at any age[22]:

- Cherish your choices and maintain control of your own life.
- Commit yourself to your passions in work and love—and embrace the conflicts and juggling involved.
- Do more than one thing well. Work at creating and maintaining flexibility.
- Don't be afraid of real intimacy with family, friends, and confidants. "Besides purpose, the research shows, ties of intimacy are the most important guarantee of a vital, long life."
- Risk being yourself, who you really are. Healthy people become more authentic as they age.
- Pay attention to what's going on—the changes in your body and the outside world, the feelings of those you love and those with whom you work.
- Risk new things, risk new ways, risk failing, risk mistakes, risk pain.
- Use technologies and medical advances if they enhance or sustain your life—but beware those that take choice away from you.
- Become a part of the changing community, and work to remain an active part of the mainstream of that community. This helps you to fill your time with valid purposes and projects.

- Live it all. Be open to all that life hands you: "the pains, disasters, surprises, unexpected openings and grace notes, detours, losses."

Step 5: Renew romance and restore a realistic, pleasurable sexual relationship. The information outlined above can help you to protect and maintain a crucial element in making your marriage resilient—your friendship. Equally important for a lifelong, happy marriage is to keep your romance alive.

Sex and romance are the most misunderstood, misrepresented, and neglected aspects of long-term marriage. Fortunately, the truth about life-long romance and later-life sex is far more reassuring and liberating than the mythology.

Myth: Menopause for women and advancing age for men inevitably lead to discomfort with sex, impotence, and eventual loss of interest in sex.

Truth: Most women do *not* lose interest in sex after menopause. In fact, many women report an upswing in their interest in sex in their sixties. Clearly, the various medical treatments currently available are wonderfully effective in countering the vaginal changes that come with menopause. Further, the 1992 National Institutes of Health's *Consensus Conference Statement on Impotence*[23] reported that fewer than 25 percent of men over sixty have erectile dysfunctions severe enough to preclude any intercourse at all. Of those who do, more than 50 percent are suffering the sexual side effects of medications or illnesses, many of which are reversible.

Myth: Sexual boredom is inevitable during the second half of marriage.

Truth: In truth, most long-term couples do not suffer from sexual boredom. Psychologist Bernard D. Starr interviewed nearly 1,000 elderly men and women about their sex lives. In the *Starr and Weiner Report on Sex and Sexuality in the Mature Years*, the researchers claimed that three fourths of elderly Americans who are sexually active say their lovemaking has improved with time.[24]

Myth: If you love each other enough, your lovemaking frequency will increase when your kids leave home, and will not decline as you age.

Truth: There's mixed news here. First, as explained by Eric Pfeiffer, M.D., the renowned geriatrician from the Center for the Study of Aging at the Duke University Medical Center, one in six of us will be even more interested in sex as we age. Why? Because a combination of physical changes that come with aging combine with the psychological phenomena of the midlife crossover to make us better lovers.

As men age, their ejaculatory demand lessens, and they need more foreplay, more tactile stimulation, and more time to become physically aroused—and all of this matches women's style of relating sexually. Plus, men become more open to intimacy of various flavors. At the same time, the midlife crossover compels an aging woman to become more comfortable being assertive and more likely to initiate sex, a change that is quite liberating for men.

But this information needs to be put into a realistic context. An aging man's newfound openness to intimacy, an aging woman's renewed assertiveness, and the freedom and privacy that a couple finds when their nest empties combine to make for a more enjoyable and comfortable sex life, but this does not always translate into increased frequency of intercourse. Rather, it appears that the reports of increased sexual pleasure with age take on various forms for different couples. Let us elaborate.

The MacArthur Foundation survey asked respondents "Over the past six months, on average, how often have you had sex with someone?" Of the age group fifty-five to sixty-four, responses were as follows[10]:

	Men	Women
Two or more times a week	18%	9%
Once a week	23%	13%
Two or three times a month	22%	16%
Once a month	9%	9%
Less often than once a month	14%	9%
Never or not at all	15%	44%

In contrast, 32 percent of both male and female respondents in the thirty-five to forty-four age range claimed to have sex two or more times a week. These statistics clearly suggest that aging does, indeed, affect the frequency of sexual activity. However, only 17 percent of women over sixty say that intercourse is necessary for good sex.

Further, the MacArthur study dispelled the myth that married couples enjoy a kind of sexual renaissance when the last child leaves home. In fact, the sexual frequency statistics for couples aged thirty-five to forty-four (most of whom are assumed to still have children at home) are virtually identical to those of the couples aged forty-five to fifty-four, the typical age of nest-emptying.

Our point is to encourage you to be realistic about the tasks that face you as you age: Build your friendship, learn to be more open and expressive in how you relate to each other physically, and deepen your intimacy—regardless of how frequently you have sexual intercourse.

Myth: Aging persons feel uncomfortable with their loss of youthful beauty.

Truth: People who age well find a refreshing liberation in learning to accept, rather than struggle with, their bodies. They move beyond shallow evaluations, to a deeper, more soulful and passionate understanding of themselves and each other. No longer are they held prisoner to unrealistic expectations of physical beauty. Betty Friedan explains it this way:

"As the years go by, warmth and curiosity, ease in relating to people, intelligence and imagination, wit and sense of irony all become far more important than looks in making up the package of attributes that people appreciate about you."[22(p6)]

One of the women interviewed by Friedan succinctly explained the liberation that comes with aging well:

"You become more whole, you put it all together—the mistakes and triumphs, the pain and sadness and joy—and you stop stewing over what your mother or father didn't do when you were 6, or over your big nose or thick ankles. You become *comfortable* with yourself, with the way you look. You don't care so much what other people think. You become a truth-teller."[13]

Final Words

Whether dealing with the empty nest, midlife issues, retirement, or the second half of marriage, healthy medical couples follow the advice that is captured in a simple saying: "No Martyrs and No Spectators."

You must stay aware *as a couple*. You have to adapt to changing partners' needs as a *couple*, and do so without either of you violating important aspects of your fundamental sense of self. Furthermore, you must do your questioning and changing *within* the marriage, continuing to make room in your private sphere for your spouse. Neither of you should be a bystander. Instead, stand *together* as you watch the answers to midlife questioning create new horizons that define a different way of living *as a couple.*

The second half of marriage can be a time of renewal for medical couples; a time to renew your teamwork, your friendship, and your romance as you take turns going through your respective midlife questioning. Face marriage's hard battles and you will grow closer and more in love in the process. If you do so, you will become one of those "wise couples" whom younger people secretly aspire to emulate.

If you know such people, observe them. Ask their advice. Encourage them to tell you stories about their marriage. They have much to teach, and you will benefit from their wisdom.

If you are such a couple, be generous in your dealings with the next generation. More than ever, medical families need to help each other. The world is generally ignorant of the unique challenges and stresses you face. If you are to stay the course, you must create safe passage for each other.

References

1. Goldberg JR. The new frontier: marriage and family therapy with aging families. *Fam Ther News.* 1992;23:14.

2. Pasko T, Seidman B. *Physician Characteristics and Distribution in the US: 1999 Edition.* Chicago, Ill: American Medical Association; 1999. See: Table B-3: Federal and Nonfederal Physicians by Age and Specialty, December 31, 1997 (Male); 52. Table B-4: Federal and Nonfederal Physicians by Age and Specialty, December 31, 1997 (Female); 53.

3. Robb N. Interest in physician-buyout packages grows as more doctors contemplate retirement. *CMAJ.* 1997;156:882-888.

4. Deane B. *Getting Ready for a Great Retirement.* Colorado Springs, Colo: NavPress; 1992:1.

5. Adapted from: Gabbard GO, Menninger RW. *Medical Marriages.* Washington, DC: American Psychiatric Press, Inc; 1988.

6. Saluter AF. *Marital Status and Living Arrangements.* Washington, DC: US Department of Commerce, Economics and Statistics Administration, Bureau of the Census; May 1991. Also see: Aquilino WS. The likelihood of parent-adult child coresidence: effects of family structure and parental characteristics. *J Marriage Fam.* 1990;52:405-419.

7. Simons D, Tiley K. Aging population and their families need sensitive consultation by family therapists. *Fam Ther News.* 1990;21:8-9.

8. Hargrave T, Anderson T. *Finishing Well: Aging and Reparation in the Intergenerational Family.* New York, NY: Brunner/Mazel; 1992.

9. Arp D, Arp C. *The Second Half of Marriage.* Grand Rapids, Mich: Zondervan Publishing House; 1996.

10. Mroczek DK, Kolarz CM. The effect of age on positive and negative affect: a developmental perspective on happiness. *J Pers Soc Psychol.* 1998;75:1333-1349.

11. Groneck S, Patterson RD. *Human Aging II: An Eleven-Year Biomedical and Behavioral Study.* US Public Health Service Monograph. Washington, DC: Government Printing Office; 1971.

12. Gutmann D. *Reclaimed Powers: Toward a New Psychology of Men and Women in Later Life.* New York, NY: McGraw-Hill; 1987.

13. For a thoughtful discussion about a woman's development at midlife, see: Friedan B. *The Fountain of Age.* New York, NY: Simon and Schuster; 1993.

14. Halpern R. *Quiet Desperation: The Truth About Successful Men.* New York, NY: Warner Books; 1988.

15. Pittman F. *Man Enough: Fathers, Sons, and the Search for Masculinity.* New York, NY: GP Putnam & Sons; 1993:15-16.

16. Robb N. Interest in physician-buyout packages grows as more doctors contemplate retirement. *CMAJ.* 1997;156:882-888.

17. Moser RH. On retirement. *Ann Intern Med.* 1997;127:159-161.

18. Merrill R, Austrom MG, Zhou H, Hendrie HC. Retirement from orthopaedic surgery. *J Bone Joint Surg.* 1999;81:414-418.

19. DeFries Z. Identity matters (or does it?). *JAMA.* 1998;279:1331.

20. McNeill RW. Retirement from orthodontics: financial and psychosocial preparation and adaptation. *Am J Orthod Dentofacial Orthop.* 1999;115:283-287.

21. Rowe JW, Kahn RL. Human aging: usual and successful. *Science.* 1987;237:143-149.

22. Friedan B. How to live longer, better, wiser. *Parade.* March 20, 1994:4-6.
23. National Institutes of Health. Impotence: Consensus Conference development conference statement; December 7-9, 1992. *Int J Impotence Res.* 1993;5:181-284.
24. Starr BD. *Starr and Weiner Report on Sex and Sexuality in the Mature Years.* New York, NY: Stein & Day; 1981.

Further Reading

Regarding family dynamics in the last stage of a parent's life:

Hargrave T, Anderson T. *Finishing Well: Aging and Reparation in the Intergenerational Family.* New York, NY: Brunner/Mazel; 1992.

Anderson D. The quest for meaningful old age. *Fam Ther Networker.*, July/August 1988:17-24.

Montalvo B, Thompson RF. Conflicts in the caregiving family. *Fam Ther Networker.* July/August 1988:31-35.

Nowitz L. A new profession for an aging society: a week in the life of a geriatric care manager. *Fam Ther Networker.* July/August 1988:36-40.

Halpern J. The reluctant caretaker: a son reaches out to his distant mother. *Fam Ther Networker.* July/August 1988:43-46.

Halpern J. *Helping Your Aging Parents: A Practical Guide for Adult Children.* New York, NY: McGraw-Hill; 1987.

For information on the MacArthur Foundation study on middle age:

New study finds middle age is prime of life. *New York Times.* February 16, 1999.

Forget the age-old myths: midlife is a place to be. *USA Today.* February 16, 1999.

For information on physicians and retirement:

Quick HE, Moen P. Gender, employment, and retirement quality: a life course approach to the differential experiences of men and women. *J Occup Health Psychol.* 1998;3:44-64.

Baker FM, Warren BH, Muraida J, Muraida G. A survey of retirement planning by Texas psychiatrists. *J Geriatr Psychiatry Neurol.* 1993;6:14-19.

Gaker FM. Retirement planning by black psychiatrists. *J Geriat Psychiatry Neurol.* 1994;7:184-188.

Gall TL, Evans DR, Howard J. The retirement adjustment process: changes in the well-being of male retirees across time. *J Gerontol, B Psychol Sci Soc Sci.* 1997;52:110-117.

Lee J, Lenzmeier T, Booulger J, Buck J, Bergeron D, Hill TJ. Retirement of senior physicians in rural Minnesota: factors influencing physicians' plans to retire. *Minn Med.* 1995;78:21-25.

Mandell H. Physicians' retirement. *Conn Med.* 1995;59:351-353.

Miscall BG, Tompkins RK, Greenfield LJ. ACS survey explores retirement and the surgeon. *Bull Am Coll Surg.* 1996;81:18-25.

Seim HC, Mitchell JE. Life after medical practice: a retirement profile of Minnesota physicians. *Minn Med.* 1995;79:27-30.

Virshup B, Coombs RH. Physicians' adjustment to retirement. *West J Med.* 1993;158:142-144.

Weiss SS, Kaplan EH, Flanagan CH Jr. Aging and retirement: a difficult issue for individual psychoanalysts and organized psychoanalysis. *Bull Menninger Clin.* 1997;61:469-480.

Weisman AD. The physician in retirement: transition and opportunity. *Psychiatry.* 1996;59:298-306.

Ward NO, Pratt LW. Otolaryngologists older than 60 years: results of and reflections on survey responses from 865 colleagues regarding retirement. *Arch Otol Head Neck Surg.* 1999;125:263-268.

Regarding Sex and Aging:

Rosenthal S. *Sex Over 40.* Los Angeles, Calif: Jeremy P. Tarcher, Inc; 1987.
McCarthy B, McCarthy E. *Couple Sexual Awareness: Building Sexual Happiness.* New York, NY: Carrol & Graf Publishers; 1998.

Rossi A. *Sexuality Across the Life Course.* Chicago, Ill: University of Chicago Press; 1999.

Chapter 8

You, Me, and Us: What's the Difference?

If there is beauty in the character, there will be harmony in the home.

—Chinese Proverb

So you got married in a haze of romanticism. You enjoyed a number of pretty good or pretty wonderful years. Then you met with disappointment and frustration, settled into power struggling, got into disillusionment, and ended up at an impasse. To top it all off, a number of crises probably bombarded you along the way.

Don't despair. What's important is what happens next.

Unfortunately, what happens next for many medical couples is not so great. Some marriages end in an uproar of anger and dismay. Other couples stay married, resigned to the notion that the romance is gone. They live in quiet pain and longing and give up the hope of renewed passion. Research suggests that medical couples tend to remain married, whether or not they are happy in their marriages.[1]

There is an exciting alternative. You *can* navigate your relationship through these rocky times without doing permanent damage, and you *can* keep your passion alive while you are at it. In fact, these same struggles that ruin many marriages can forge a greater strength, respect, and love. It depends on whether you can accomplish two things: differentiation, *and* an honest evaluation of the intimacy factor in your relationship.

Declaring Your Differences

If your marriage is going to grow, you periodically have to allow yourselves to grow apart—at least a little. Here we are referring to what marriage and family therapists call differentiation, which has to do with clarifying where one of you leaves off and the other begins. Differentiation moves you from the "two of us together will make one whole person" mythology into a more mature appreciation of the two unique individuals that you are and a realistic understanding of the possibilities for your marriage. Through differentiation, you help each other out of the starstruck one-true-love fantasies (and the strangling, drowning quagmire created by power struggling and disillusionment) and into a fresh, mature love and romance.

Differentiation is a process, not an event. Healthy couples first work to create it and then cooperate to maintain it by taking three steps, each of which is easier said than done.

Differentiation Step 1: Accepting the Limits of Your Power to Change Each Other. No matter how much you do to or for each other, the fundamental truth remains: There is a clear point at which one of you leaves off and the other begins as a distinct, independent person. You'll take a giant step out of power struggling and disillusionment when you shift from trying desperately to change each other to focusing on what each of you can do to make the relationship a more comfortable place for each other (given who the two of you have become).

Differentiation Step 2: Recognizing the Different Flavors of Emptiness. To be human is to struggle with essential aloneness. For ages, theologians and philosophers have cautioned us to beware that this fact will sometimes leave us feeling empty. No matter who we are or how deserving of nurturing, we will sometimes be reminded that we are not now, and never have been, the center of anyone else's universe. Yet, in marriage, we each seem to believe, "if only my one true love weren't so hardheaded, he or she could make *me* the exception to this universal rule."

The second step in differentiation involves understanding the sources of the painful feelings that you sometimes experience and controlling the tendency to blame each other when you are hurting. This is difficult to do when, on a given day, it seems clear that your discomfort *is* all about your marriage. But remember that your relationship is not the only part of your life that generates emotions. Emotional pain comes from many sources: our essential aloneness in the world, the drain of an overwhelming lifestyle, and the memories of past struggles that have nothing to do with our current relationships, to name but a few.

As the old saying goes: "You always hurt the one you love." Human nature compels us to displace our frustrations by projecting blame for our pain onto our most convenient targets—loved ones. Loving couples work hard to recognize when pain or discomfort is coming from nonrelationship factors, and to stop the pain from getting dumped into their marriage. This can only be done by taking the third step in differentiation.

Differentiation Step 3: Blocking Displacement and Projections. High-powered people often live out an interesting paradox, the "Dr. Jekyll and Mr. Hyde" displacement of anger and projection of blame. We go off to work, where we tolerate an endless bombardment of stress, all the while storing our frustration. Then we come home and act as though these people whom we have hardly seen all day (our family) are the *sole* cause of our irritation, frustration, and fatigue. Let's look at how this might occur, from the inside.

Displacement. High-powered people take charge of their lives. We use our skills and coping strength to get things done well. However, in the process, we do *not* take very good care of *ourselves*. Busy people often do a poor job of managing themselves in relationships. We can manage *other* people, but sell out *ourselves*. Research has shown that, as a group, physicians tend to be sensitive, conscientious people who are dedicated to caretaking activities and who have difficulty giving themselves permission to set limits in responding to the expectations of others.[2,3] Our consulting experiences with medical groups have repeatedly suggested that physicians also tend to be conflict avoiders.

As an illustration, pretend that you are watching a split screen showing two videotapes: on screen 1 are the activities and interactions from a week in the life of a typical high-powered person. Simultaneously, screen 2 is showing a videotape of that person's thoughts and feelings as he or she goes through the episodes showing on the first screen.

On screen 1 the person looks strong and effective. But screen 2's glimpses into that person's inner experiences would suggest that this dynamo often behaves in a strangely unassertive manner. While screen 1 showed a powerful—even intimidating—person, screen 2 reveals a person with ruffled feathers, unsalved hurts, and unexpressed frustrations, as evidenced by thoughts like:

"What the hell! I might as well do it myself!"

"Well, what can you expect from other people?"

"That hurt. But that's just the way he is."

"Got to go on."

"I'm too busy to deal with this."

In short, screen 2 shows an upwardly moving graph of tension as the physician simply goes numb and keeps performing.

In this way, many of us accumulate tension. We arrive home with a storm of static electricity inside, looking for a "lightning rod" to strike. A misplaced word by a loved one, a rejected overture of affection, or a spilled glass of milk can serve as a catalyst. This is *displacement*.

Projection. A related psychological "trick" is called *projection*. In its most obvious form, projection involves selectively perceiving our unexpressed "bad-self" traits when we look at our spouse. Our loved one's face and voice become associated with one side of our most complicated internal splits.

To make matters worse, we get each other to cooperate in projective processes by accusing, picking at, and prodding our partner into revealing those parts of himself or herself that match our own unexpressed self. This is called *projective identification*.

These battles blur the boundaries of where one of you leaves off and the other begins. During the stages of intoxicating infatuation with our one true love, we identify with each other's positive projections—our "good self." As we settle into power struggling and disillusionment, we shift into projecting and identifying with each other's "bad self."

As a relationship settles into an enactment of our internal psychological struggles, we move away from our partner. Doing so creates the illusion of having resolved the unresolved internal issues that are fueling the projective process in the first place.

The more narcissistic you are, the greater your internal psychological splitting. The more split you are, the more self-focused you are likely to be. The more self-focused you are, the more likely you are to project and displace your discomfort onto your mate. The more you project and displace, the more likely you are to pursue and distance in a desperate effort to find comfort from all of the above. The more this does not work, the more discomfited you will become, perpetuating even a greater degree of self-focusing. We treat many couples who are living their lives on this not-so-merry-go-round.

Allowing your relationship to revolve around projections that are fueled by your own ambivalence about "unacceptable" aspects of yourself can render you a lifetime member of the Miserably Married Club. Beware of what psychiatrist Robert Beavers calls striking "the unholy bargain":

> You take one-half of my ambivalence and I'll take the other half of yours. Neither of us will experience an internal conflict and both of our anxiety levels will drop; our self-image will seem clearer. The only unfortunate side effect is that we will fight like hell for 40 years.[4]

Variations of the theme of projection. Projection takes many forms in intimate relationships. In fact, most scholars in the field of marriage and family therapy agree that it is impossible to avoid falling into at least pockets of projection during the course of a romance. This makes sense. To join as closely as is needed in order to make a life together, two people are bound to at least periodically get confused about where one leaves off and the other begins. Each begins to believe that the other is the cause of both their positive and their negative inner experiences.

Even if you had a happy childhood and a prior string of nurturing, loving relationships, you will try to shape your current romance into something that feels familiar. Unfortunately, this process will probably cloud your ability to experience the person with whom you are trying to negotiate a relationship.

We are particularly prone to blur psychological boundaries whenever our current life circumstances mimic old, unresolved issues. Robert Beavers points out:

> The more a member of a couple has been raised in a family where unresolved conflict has festered and impaired family functioning, the more difficulty that person has in resolving his own individual ambivalence about significant relationships.[4]

We offer a few case examples in hopes of clarifying how projection and projective identification look, feel, and sound in marriage.

Marvin and Marsha

Marvin, an obstetrician-gynecologist, was referred to counseling because his employer's quality-management committee received complaints from five women that he had made lewd or cruel comments to them during his delivery of medical care. His story shows how projection can come from one's internal conflicts and how it can ruin a marriage.

Marvin was reared in a sexually oppressive environment. He was never comfortable with his range of sexual feelings. He had what psychologists often call a "mother-whore" complex, viewing women in black-or-white terms. The "good" women of the world were the all-nurturing Madonnas who deserved respect and admiration for their virtue and for their maternal nature. The "bad" women—the ones that Marvin spent hours fantasizing about with his hidden pornography collection—stirred feelings of intrigue and repulsion.

Problems developed in Marvin's marriage as he projected his own psychological split about sexuality onto his wife, Marsha. At first, Marvin assigned the role of Madonna to his wife. He saw her as the mother of his children and his own nurturer.

These perceptions of Marsha were the foundation of Marvin's love and commitment to her. But these same perceptions led to problems as both Marvin and Marsha grew bored with their marriage. Marvin was tired of having such a "homely" wife. He sought out other relationships in which he expressed his playful, passionate side. Of course, in his distorted way of thinking, Marvin saw the women in these affairs as being

"bad." Predictably, they became the targets of the repulsion he associated with his own sexuality. He typically ended an affair with some act of
scornful cruelty.

In contrast to the distorted image that Marvin held of her, Marsha
was anything but "homely." She was a nurturing caretaker but also a
vibrant, attractive, and intelligent woman who had a quick wit and a
wonderful spirit of playfulness.

Marsha, too, grew bored with the marriage. She tired of Marvin's discomfort and disapproval whenever she tried to get him to loosen up and
have sexual fun. He seemed intrigued and aroused if she acted sexually
aggressive and even periodically brought home sexy negligees as an invitation for them to "play dress-up." These fun and exciting times were a
"recess" from their typical roles and responsibilities.

Inevitably, however, after a period of sexual playfulness, Marvin
would withdraw. He would launch into work, become numb, unavailable, and irritable, and eventually strike out at Marsha with a barrage of
criticism.

Marsha became suspicious when she stumbled upon Marvin's stash
of pornography. She began to covertly keep tabs on his activities and followed Marvin one night as he was supposedly going back to the hospital
to finish rounds. Instead, he drove to a bar that featured nude dancers.

Expecting a barrage of justifications and rationalizations, Marsha
confronted her husband. To her surprise, Marvin simply apologized. He
admitted that his interest in pornography had created a lifelong struggle,
and he vowed to rid his life of the problem.

The crisis blew over, but the projective process that was lurking
beneath the surface festered. In the heat of honest discussions following
Marsha's discoveries, she admitted her boredom with the marriage. This
was done in the tone of, "Come on, Marvin. Don't leave me out! I'm not
the prude you think I am. I might be more interested in playing sexual
games than you imagine. You don't have to go to strangers. Let's you and
me play!"

For a while, Marsha and Marvin began rewriting the sexual part of
their relationship. For months they enjoyed a renewed focus on their sex
life. They played sexual games and watched sexy movies together. They
made love in new ways. They talked about their sexual fantasies and
enacted those that they thought would be fun. In short, they expanded
the boundaries of sex in their relationship.

Then they collided with another pocket of Marvin's projections. He
began accusing Marsha of going through "some kind of midlife crisis"
and shamed her about "dressing in ways that call attention to yourself."
He sulked following any social occasion; he would become sarcastic and
accusatory, saying, "You sure seemed to be enjoying moving your ass a
lot when you were dancing tonight. It looked to me like you were trying
to put on a show. Who were you performing for?"

In a renewed flurry of projection, Marvin honed in on Marsha's vul-
nerability. Based on events that had actually transpired—sexual games
the two of them had orchestrated, sexual fantasies that his wife had
trusted him enough to share, requests for change in their sex life that
Marsha had lovingly made—Marvin constructed an image of his wife
that shifted her from Madonna to whore. Tragically, this man's selective
perceptions and projections led to the demise of the marriage. Just as he
had done in his affairs, Marvin cruelly and scornfully cast his wife aside,
proclaiming her "a whore in disguise."

Several Brief Examples of Projection.

- A father who had a painful adolescence becomes atypically cruel to his children when they show their own adolescent joys and enthusiasm.

Underlying projection: His kids' successes and their comfortable lifestyle (created, in large part, by his own efforts) stir unresolved feelings of loss for the father.

- A woman who did not get her fair share of nurturing when she was young tends to overwork and overworry. The more fatigued she grows, the more she accuses her husband of being inattentive.

Underlying projection: Her husband becomes the "lightning rod" for the stored pain that comes from her own underdeveloped capacity for self-nurturing.

- A man who never felt masculine enough or good about his appearance obsesses about whether or not his wife is gaining weight.

Underlying projection: His own self-doubts get projected in the form of criticizing his wife about her appearance.

- A woman who was taught to fear her own impulsivity lives in fear that her husband might develop a drinking problem. She obsessively monitors how many beers he consumes over a weekend and how many cocktails he drinks at a party. In truth, the man doesn't drink much.

Underlying projection: The woman's internal conflicts about control versus loss of control now have an interpersonal vehicle through which they can be expressed.

The possibilities here are endless. There exists an unfortunate paradox in marriage. The very ways of interacting that create growth in your relationship can stir the most primitive distress. Then the defenses of projection and displacement get stirred in response to your anxiety about being in this new territory. Unfortunately, while these defense mechanisms give you momentary comfort, they serve to push you back into old, painfully familiar ways of interacting with each other. Unless they are controlled, projection and displacement will sabotage your attempts to renegotiate your relationship contract.

Differentiation, a first step that can lead out of disillusionment, requires clarifying psychological boundaries. To differentiate successfully, you must do three things:

- Accept the limits of your power to change each other.
- Clarify your various flavors of emptiness.
- Block the tendencies to displace anger and project blame.

These steps help you clarify your individuality. Next, you must honestly evaluate your relationship patterns.

Evaluation

All your feelings and conflicts are not always due to psychological hang-ups. Sometimes your emotions are simply a reaction to what is or is not happening *right now*. Psychological hocus-pocus doesn't explain everything about anything. Most of what has to be negotiated to keep your marriage alive will be what is happening *between* you, *not* what is veiled in a shroud of psychological complexity that began in your childhood. Age-old psychological issues might complicate the negotiations, but here-and-now issues must be attended to nonetheless.

Systems Resist Changing

Even when dealing with a relationship problem that *is* confined to the present, solving it can be confusing. Why is change in marriage so hard to pull off even when you both agree that a new way of dealing with each other would be better?

Growth in marriage is complicated by a simple fact: Relationships *themselves* resist changing.

Your perceptions of each other and your ways of interacting become habits. Remember: Change requires adjusting and therefore is stressful. Even if you decide that changing is in your best interest, your old relationship stress positions will tend to keep you acting and perceiving in ways that feel familiar.

This fact alone can sabotage well-intentioned efforts to grow more healthy. The awkwardness that comes with changing old relationship habits can override the payoffs for making any change. Behaviors such as arguing, smoking, drinking, using drugs, overworking, or acting out a certain attitude about sex can become integral parts of a relationship. We remain stuck in the familiar roles and rituals that organize the relationship even when we dislike the consequences.

What Will Happen if *You* Change?

Even though we believe that changing yourself is the best way to increase the odds that your relationship will change, let's not ignore the obvious. If it is to grow, the *relationship* must change. Changes of any sort create a period of awkwardness and tension. Once you change, negative feelings last until you become familiar with the new relationship that you are putting in place. You must accept that awkwardness.

In intimate relationships, awkwardness may be perceived as a sign that the other partner is trying to punish us through withdrawal or some other form of rejection. If this happens, you are likely to recycle back into power struggling instead of working as a team.

James and Gretchen Jacobson experienced this sort of relationship tension.

The Jacobsons

The Jacobsons were hard-driving individuals who were partners in every way: They shared responsibilities for their home and family, and they each thrived in their respective medical careers—Gretchen's in neurology, James's in internal medicine.

The Jacobsons were proud that they worked hard but also found time to play hard. They regularly took "nights off," enjoying expensive wines, talking about their life and relationship, seducing each other. All went well until Gretchen's liver problems forced them to reexamine their lifestyle.

Gretchen decided to quit drinking, and James volunteered to cut out alcohol as well. Within six months, Gretchen's liver function tests indicated improvement, but her marriage showed signs of strain.

In this new chapter of their relationship, the Jacobsons plowed through their weeks, absorbed in the stress of their high-powered lives but not connected in that old romantic, passionate way that had always been their main source of rejuvenation. One obvious problem was that once they stopped drinking, the Jacobsons also curtailed their romancing. Gretchen explained it this way: "The truth is that James and I courted each other for eighteen years with those 'nights off' filled with drinking and talking late into the evening. Since our medical school days, we always had the same pattern: We worked like maniacs for a few days, then escaped quickly with the help of a few drinks or a couple of bottles of good wine. That became our courtship ritual.

"When we stopped drinking, we also stopped our courtship. All we do now is work. I sort of miss the alcohol, but I miss the romance even more. I just never realized what a habit we were in and how hard it is to get used to a new way of taking time out to be with each other."

James explained it somewhat differently: "I feel like Gretchen is angry with me. I think she blames me for her health problems. You see, she never really wanted me to go into private practice. She worries about the future of private enterprise in medicine and is really security focused when it comes to money. She thinks that academic medicine is a safer bet. She said from the get-go that life would be too stressful if I went into practice mainly because of her fears about money. I was the one that steamrolled her into going along with this deal. Now I think she blames me for the stress that affected her health.

"Maybe I am to blame. I don't know. I just did what I thought was best for me and therefore for us. The opportunity was there, and I thought it wise to jump on it.

"But I hate the way she is withdrawing from me. It's like she's saying, 'You see what the stress almost did to me? I had to drink to cope. Now this damned life we are living leaves me so tired and worried, I don't have any energy left over for you.'

"I hate this. I feel guilty. I feel somehow responsible. I also feel angry with Gretchen. I don't know what to do."

The Jacobsons profited from open discussion about what was happening between them. They reconnected as they put words to their fears, their regrets, their awkwardness, and to the longing they felt for each other. Their struggle ended when they evaluated themselves and clearly communicated what they were thinking, feeling, and needing from each other.

Such dialogue led the Jacobsons into a three-month experiment: They decided to once again begin taking regular nights off for romance, this time without the alcohol. In this way, they recreated their most familiar vehicle for communicating, and James's fears that Gretchen was secretly seething with anger toward him were put to rest. Even though they both admitted feeling awkward, like they missed the familiar feeling of their old intoxicated way of "relaxing," they were eventually able to replace their old pattern with a new, more healthy version of romance.

The Jacobsons saved their marriage with their honesty. Other couples, like Hal and Toni in the following case example, complicated their efforts to renegotiate their relationship contract with a strange form of dishonesty that holds the relationship together.

Hal and Toni

Hal was a dynamic, successful attorney who was the evident head of the household. He ruled his children and wife, Toni, with an iron fist. He controlled how they spent money, how they spent their time on weekends, whom they associated with, and much of what was said during dinnertime conversations.

Hal was in control of most aspects of his marriage and family life, except one: He periodically had temper tantrums triggered by normal levels of family stress. At such times, he verbally abused his children.

Even during relatively calm times, Hal generally felt awkward and clumsy dealing with his children. This was a secret that only Toni knew, and it became her most powerful lever of control in her private dealings with Hal. He was embarrassed by his temper and by his ineptness as a parent.

But Hal's was not the only secret in this marriage. Toni, too, was vulnerable to knowledge held only by her spouse. Although she was a pediatrician "who ought to know better" (her words), Toni had been bulimic for five years. She regularly binged on high-carbohydrate foods and then purged by vomiting or taking laxatives. Hal learned of Toni's problem when he unexpectedly arrived home one day and discovered her gorging herself on sweets.

This was a fact that only Hal knew and was only discussed in the heat of a certain kind of argument. If Toni shamed Hal for his outbursts with their children, he broke their tacit agreement that they would cooperate in denying Toni's problem. With a bullying bravado, he was usually able to end their fights with a threat that frightened Toni into withdrawal: "All right. If it's as awful around here as you say it is—all because of me—let's call a therapist tomorrow. I'll go if you will. But only if we agree to tell the shrink the whole damned truth. I'm not the only one around here who has problems."

Telling the Truth

Denial requires cooperation. It is dangerous to cooperate with each other in denying emotional or physical problems. Doing so creates a weak spot in the foundation of your relationship. The weak spot is created not only by the problems per se but by the fact that the relationship becomes part of what perpetuates the problems. Sooner or later most people decide to face the truth about themselves. If your relationship promotes self-deception, when the time of reckoning comes, the relationship will be deemed a major contributor to—rather than a solution to—your struggles.

In truth, most of us do have some unhealthy habit or growth-limiting ethic that is protected by the "rules" of our most intimate relationships. Honestly evaluating whether or not you have some form of unhealthy cooperation or struggle going on in your relationship is at once interesting and frightening.

The possibilities here are endless. For example, the "rules" of your relationship might dictate that you repress your emotions, act in racially prejudiced ways, believe only in a certain religion or political philosophy, associate only with certain people, or engage in a specific unhealthy behavior in order to fit into the relationship.

Our intention is not to moralize here. We are simply posing two important questions:

- What are the behaviors and attitudes that organize *your* relationship?
- Do *you* want to continue to organize your life and your relationship in these ways?

The following exercises are designed to help you answer these questions.

The Behaviors and Attitudes of Our Relationship

Think of the many behaviors and attitudes that organize your relationship. Force yourself to think broadly. Truthfully examine how you are living and the many roles that you have assigned to each other and have assumed in your intimate teamwork. List several of these behaviors or attitudes.

(To clarify this exercise, see the following examples from the case of Hal and Toni.)

Behaviors	Attitudes
1. Toni's bulimia.	1. Hal's anger is accepted.
2. Hal's verbal abuse.	2. Toni's bulimia is denied.
3. Hal's control over social life.	3. We agree that certain types of people are not worth knowing.
Our Behaviors	**Our Attitudes**

Next, imagine how your relationship would change if you stopped participating in each of these behaviors or attitudes. How would you feel? How do you imagine your partner would react? What would you have to change if you stopped this behavior or changed this attitude? What relationship patterns would be affected by such changes?

Clarifying Your Authentic Self

Your responses to the above exercise can form an outline for a very important process. These responses can help you begin to clarify your authentic self amid the roles that you have assumed within your marriage and family.

If you had difficulty pinpointing behaviors and attitudes that organize your relationship *and* thwart your authenticity, you are probably relatively comfortable in your relationship. If so, you are fortunate, and chances are you authentically express yourself within your relationship.

But if you pinpointed ways that you are being inauthentic in order to fit into a relationship pattern, then you face an important decision: Either get honest with yourself and your partner—even if this means facing the heat of conflict—or run the high risk of growing resentful in the relationship and gradually distancing from your partner.

Evaluating Your Relationship Teamwork

How are you doing in your relationship teamwork? Is your love, appreciation, and respect for each other enhanced by the ways that you cooperate in creating your life's territory, or are you struggling with each other as you react to the changes and challenges that face you?

Use the following lists to examine yourselves. Check the items that apply to you or someone you love. You will notice that with the omission of those items that obviously refer to romance, this same list can be used to assess any family relationship. You might benefit from doing this exercise several times, noting what applies to you and your spouse, to you and each of your children, or to you and other selected family members.

Signs of Positive Relationship Teamwork

- You openly and frequently talk about your life: your respective dreams, fantasies, fears, pressures, victories, and disappointments.
- Without nagging or policing each other, you encourage each other to stick to your plans to better yourselves.
- You offer help to each other when motivation to live more healthily begins to sag.
- No one is victimized by the choices you make as you try to take better care of yourself.
- You help each other make time to take care of yourselves.
- You encourage each other to reward yourselves for this healthier way of living.
- You allow each other to express strong emotions.
- You accept that relationships, just like individuals, grow and change and that you therefore must periodically alter your expectations and ways of relating to each other in order to adjust to new ways of being together.
- You are honest with each other about what you think, feel, need, and want.

- You are flexible in your roles as you deal with the tasks and responsibilities facing your family.
- When you have conflicts, you listen, empathize, and compromise with each other.
- You privately and publicly express respect and appreciation for each other.
- You avoid using power-struggle tactics. You are direct, honest, and fair in trying to get your needs and desires met.
- You are gentle and forgiving in dealing with each other.
- You encourage and help each other develop abilities and traits that will make you more complete people.
- You try not to be driven by stress and frustration.
- Rather than clinging to the unrealistic belief that a relationship can work naturally, you accept the fact that you will have to work to keep the healing spirit of your relationship alive.
- You are able to forgive each other for mistakes.
- You are at peace with the fact that no one—no matter how good or loving they may be—is perfect.
- You regularly have fun together.
- In your marriage, you continue that "boyfriend-girlfriend" action that serves as the core of your romance. You regularly notice, court, and romance each other.
- In your marriage, you regularly let each other know that you still choose each other.

Signs of Family Struggles

Remember that families are teams. Accordingly, any member of the team can be the symptom bearer during times of stress, and any member's struggles can stress the family. If any member of a family is showing signs of struggle, one of two possibilities is likely: Either (a) that person's symptoms indicate that the family is struggling or (b) that person's struggles are likely to stress the family.

- You refuse to accept the truth if someone you love (including yourself) is going through a difficult time.
- During stressful times in your relationship, you remain ignorant about what needs to change in order to make the relationship better.
- You try to cram as much activity and action into your life as possible. You live as though you are afraid to slow down.
- Your attitude is one of persistent hostility.
- Following the onset of a stressful time, one or both of you show a prolonged exaggeration of some personality trait. For example: A typically orderly person may become compulsively neat, a typically quiet person may become withdrawn, or a typically cautious person may begin to act paranoid.
- You discount the possibility that things can improve. You act pessimistic and defeatist.
- Old relationship problems get worse under the strain of current stresses.
- As you face your tasks, responsibilities, and emotional difficulties, you rigidly lock into roles within the relationship.

• You blame or shame each other.

• You refuse to express emotion.

• In your emotional dealings with each other, you are stingy rather than nurturing and generous.

• You disagree about your definition of the tasks that face you. For example, one of you might define your current situation as a challenge and an opportunity to show strength of character, while the other sees it as a sign of defeat.

• You refuse to open up to each other for fear of upsetting the other person.

• You passively or indirectly fight back in power struggles with each other rather than directly dealing with your differences.

• You turn to another (e.g., one of your children or siblings) to gossip about each other rather than dealing directly with each other about your differences.

• Your marriage is not sexually fulfilling.

On an additional sheet of paper, add other signs of positive or negative functioning in *your* relationship.

Giving Each Other Feedback

Once you have completed the above exercises, we recommend that you do two things: First, discuss what you learned about the various ways your relationship is healthy and helpful to you. Be loving and positive. Compliment each other and elaborate on the specifics of what you like and appreciate about each other. Describe what is positive about your ways of coping as a couple and what you admire and appreciate about each other.

Next, with this same spirit of caring, discuss the relationship concerns and fears that surfaced in responding to these exercises. (Before doing so, you might want to preview the guidelines for conflict resolution in Chapter 13.) Underscore your willingness to work *with* (and not *against*) each other as you face these problems.

While you discuss these concerns, bear in mind our aforementioned advice about controlling such relationship tricks as projection of blame or displacement of anger. Remember: "The awful truth is that what is most intolerable to you about your mate is at least partially your recognition in your partner of what you cannot bear to recognize in yourself."[5]

Dare to Be You!

At the outset of the power-struggle stage of marriage, most of us fear that being too vocal about our differences might ruin our relationship. We fear that such honesty might taint our idealized love for each other.

As a marriage matures, we have to mature with it. This means taking the chance of being more honest in our self-examinations and in our conversations with each other.

When you muster the courage and the maturity to evaluate your relationship honestly and discuss your observations lovingly, you begin to differentiate. This allows you to renegotiate your relationship contract, this time in the light of mature love. In this new territory you will discover unexpected relief from your pain. You will become more familiar with two fascinating people—your partner, whom you will begin to see in a new light, and your own authentic, integrated self.

You will not find that either of you is perfect. The result is both healing and heartwarming. Give yourself permission to take better care of yourself rather than waiting for some magical "other" to make you into a more complete person. Experience your mate as a nurturing partner, not a screen onto which you have projected your good and bad fantasies about love and marriage. Begin to see your mate as someone deserving of your love and affection, even though you both accept that you cannot change each other.

As you go through this process, a new flavor of intimacy is likely to develop in your relationship. The payoff for enduring the power-struggle and disillusionment stages of marriage and for fighting to create and maintain differentiation is that your relationship becomes nurturing and affirming rather than toxic—a crucial ingredient in effective emotional management. Such a marriage is described in *Heart Illness and Intimacy: How Caring Relationships Aid Recovery:*

> Each partner now begins to appreciate the other in new ways. A renewed appreciation blossoms. But now this loving impression of the other is not viewed through the rose-colored glasses of immature and unrealistic expectations about love and marriage. Rather, couples consciously begin to examine the basic questions that underlie marriage: Do we accept the limits on how much our marriage can soothe our internal psychological struggling? Do we still choose to face the challenge of living as two separate people who work lovingly to be healing partners in this complicated but worthwhile experience of being married?[6]

References

1. Garvey M, Tuason VB. Physician marriages. *J Clin Psychiatry*. 1979;40:129-131.
2. Marcus IM. Harmony vs. discord in marriage: a view of physicians' marriages. *J La State Med Soc*. 1980;132:173-178.
3. Gabbard GO. The role of compulsiveness in the normal physician. JAMA. 1985;254:2926-2929.
4. Beavers R. *Successful Mariage: A Family Systems Approach to Couples Therapy*. New York, NY: WW Norton; 1985:30.
5. Hendrix H. *Getting the Love You Want: A Guide for Couples*. New York, NY: Harper& Row; 1990.
6. Sotile WM. *Heart Illness and Intimacy: How Caring Relationships Aid Recovery*. Baltimore, Md: Johns Hopkins University Press; 1992.

Part 3

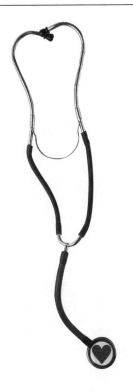

Medicine, Marriage, and Stress

Chapter 9

Flavors of Medical Marriages: Complications in the Renegotiations

The more I learn about people, the less comfortable do I feel about generalizing.

—**Irwin M. Marcus, M.D.**

The initial stages of romance for medical couples are not unique. However, marriages that revolve around a medical career (or careers) are unique in three ways:

- Your initial relationship contracts are more complex than those for other couples.
- As your relationship develops, your high-powered coping styles are especially likely to complicate the power struggle and disillusionment stages of your marriage.
- Contract renegotiation in your relationship is likely to be complicated by the unique ways that you are likely to react to relationship stresses. By the very nature of one or both of your ace-in-the-hole coping strategies, you are likely to have difficulty with the essentials of conflict resolution: empathy, validation of the other person's perspectives, patience, acceptance, and a willingness to experiment with modifying your own steps in crucial relationship dances.

What Needs to Be Done About This?

The complexity of answering this question is suggested in the following list of "Confessions of Spouses of Superachievers." Over the past twenty years, we have accumulated hundreds of descriptions of hard-driving, time-urgent, high-powered people that were given by their mates. Many of the high-powered people in question were physicians; many were spouses of physicians. A glimpse at these comments sheds light on an important first step in deciphering medical-marriage struggles—understanding how the players view the inner workings of each other and their relationship.

"My wife is the most confident-acting, insecure person I have ever known."

"For someone who is so outgoing, it is surprising how lonely and misunderstood he secretly feels."

"He has an office filled with plaques and certificates that document his accomplishments and the applause that he has gotten. But he still feels unappreciated, unrecognized, and that he has not yet proved himself. Worse yet, he seems to believe that I don't think that he has succeeded."

"The only time she seems to feel secure is right after she has received some form of recognition: after having a paper accepted for publication or when someone says something admiring to her about what kind of mother she is. But the satisfaction never lasts. She drives herself relentlessly."

"He wakes up scared in the middle of the night. Each morning, I have to give him a pep talk that lets him know what a wonderful physician he is and how important and appreciated he is. I sometimes feel like a cheerleader."

"Her rage attacks are scary to me and my kids. She would die if she knew I was telling you this. Psychiatrists aren't supposed to act this way."

"No matter how much or how well she does, she begins and ends each day by making mental notes about what she should be feeling stressed and guilty about not having yet done—she calls it her 'to do' list."

"When I hug him, he stiffens. When we make love, he either doesn't seem to know what to do or acts like a robot stuck on one speed. For a physician, he certainly is naive when it comes to sex."

"When he worked in academic medicine, he lived in fear of his chairman's criticism. Now he has his own practice, and he lives in fear of his patients' criticism."

"She gets a gleam of joy in her eye whenever she talks about any hard times that friends or relatives are going through. She's the most competitive person I know."

"Beneath all of that control lurks anxiety and chaos."

"He acts like he couldn't care less about you or what you think, but I'll guarantee you this: If you say anything negative about him, he will never *forget it, and he will* never *forgive you."*

"I just wish that she would stop torturing herself by comparing herself to everyone else."

"Comparing yourself to your siblings or peers is one thing. But he even compares himself to famous people and then feels bad about not having accomplished enough with his life."

"Relaxing makes her tense. She only acts like she's having fun if she is being stimulated in some new and different way."

"He tries to be a good dad, but his attention span is shorter than that of our children."

"If you aren't talking about him or about what he's interested in, then he grows bored and distracted."

"The woman lives in a constant state of frustration."

"He is ashamed of how prejudiced he is. The truth is that he treats black patients differently than he treats other patients."

"She condemns anybody who gets in her way as being a member of a class of undesirable people. It doesn't matter—fat, skinny, short, tall, white, black, poor, rich—if they are in her way, they are disgusting to her."

"Being with him is like walking on eggshells. You never know when you're going to take a wrong step. Then you get his anger."

"He has learned to come home at a reasonable hour, but the truth is, he feels guilty unless he is working at something that seems absolutely necessary."

"When I see him with his parents and siblings, he looks like a desperate little boy hoping to get noticed and patted on the back."

"She is the most interpersonally powerful woman that I know. But she turns into a scared little girl when she talks with her daddy."

"I used to see him as being so powerful and capable. In truth, he is a pretty boring, constrained person. He is afraid to expand his horizons. Of course, he claims that he just isn't interested in 'all that hoity-toity stuff.'"

Family relationships are the most private arenas of exposure and vulnerability for anyone, and high-powered people seem to have particular difficulty with the negative feedback and demands for compromise that are inherent in a long-term, intimate relationship. Often growth in marriage is gained at the cost of feedback that is difficult to say and to hear. No matter how loving the confrontation is, an exceptionally controlling, cognitively oriented person is likely to react with defensiveness and irritability.

We superachievers are not very fond of being confronted with our shortcomings. Furthermore, the more narcissistic we get, the more we are likely to recoil from the bearer of any less than flattering news about ourselves. Such reflexive reactions will complicate attempts to renegotiate any relationship contract.

Flavors of Medical Marriages

We believe that the coping styles that come with our busy lives can shape marital dynamics in several ways, depending on two factors: (1) the presence of Type A behavior pattern (TYABP) in one or both partners, and (2) the variant of TYABP (e.g., "hot reactor," "healthy Type A," etc.). Our own clinical observations as well as information from research literature regarding medical marriages suggest eight conceptual frameworks that help to elucidate the inner workings of medical marriages.

Eight Types of Medical Marriages

- Pattern 1: *We're a Physician: Two People, One Medical Career*
- Pattern 2: *The Physician and His Wife: Pleasing Others Even if It Kills Them*
- Pattern 3: *The Physician and Her Husband: Pleasing Others Even if It Kills Her*
- Pattern 4: *Ready, Set, Go! The Physicians and Other Dual-Career Couples*
- Pattern 5: *Chaotic Desperation: When Hot Reactors Kill the Love*
- Pattern 6: *The Island Man or Woman: When Cold Reactors Kill the Love*
- Pattern 7: *Too Mellow to Admit It*
- Pattern 8: *Using Our Good Stuff to Make It Better*

It is impossible to characterize all of the forms that medical marriages can take. Every couple is unique in their coping styles, strengths, and weaknesses. The following patterns are not mutually exclusive and are not exhaustive of all possibilities. However, we have found that these concepts have been useful to the many physicians and their loved ones whom we have had the privilege of counseling and training. We offer these descriptions in the hope that they will help you to better understand what has happened, what is happening, or what is likely to happen in your relationship.

Chapter 10

How Much Is Enough?

Male physicians tend to engage in selective recruitment in seeking a marriage partner, with the aim of finding someone who will fit into the singlemindedness of the physician's lifestyle.

—Ira D. Glick, M.D. and Jonathan F. Borus, M.D.

The first two patterns in our model revolve around struggles that occur when the male is the only physician in the marriage. In both of the patterns discussed in this chapter, a relentless quest to achieve some vaguely defined, elusive sense of personal well-being erodes marital intimacy. In the *We're a Physician: Two People, One Medical Career* pattern, a physician-husband's self-involvement drains the life out of the marriage. In *The Physician and His Wife: Pleasing Others Even if It Kills Them* pattern, marriage and family life are bombarded, not by the physician, but by his Type A wife's relentless quest to be all things to all people.

Pattern 1: We're a Physician: Two People, One Medical Career

This classic medical marital pattern is characteristic of many traditional, high-powered relationships. Here, an ambitious, career-oriented male physician and a nurturing "good mother" find each other.

Their Roles

The original marital contract explicitly states that the wife will be the nurturer and stress absorber for the couple. The physician-husband will be a hard worker whose extrafamilial involvements (like work, community activities, and avocational interests) will bring status, prestige, and stress to the marriage and family.

This arrangement works nicely for both partners, especially through the early childbearing and child-rearing years of the marriage—a stage that, despite its high levels of stress, fosters appreciation of all that the other partner is doing in the quest to create a fulfilling life. For a while, many women are satisfied with the roles that come with this marital pattern: caretaker and "junior partner." These roles conform to the socialization of many women. During the initial years of marriage, such wives often report a quiet sense of pride and dignity stemming from being all-nurturing and patient, allowing for their husbands' long hours and other demands that arise from their husbands' education, training, and work as physicians.

Until fairly recently, examples of this "junior partner" role could be found throughout the literature on medical marriages. For example, an article written by a physician spouse and published in the *Journal of the Florida Medical Association* in 1977 offered the following "pearls" of wisdom for women married to physicians:

> Being sympathetic, understanding and keeping the family hum of activity going will be greatly appreciated, but don't fail to keep the bread winner informed so that he can participate in the family circle as much as possible. . . . When children are involved, be sure that they understand at an early age the demands made on their Dad's time . . . It isn't the quantity of time with a child, but rather the quality! Too, because that special Dad might not be able to get to the store, you can help him give the children those little surprises that will light up their eyes. Just buy them and let him present them; he'll enjoy the role of "super-dad," and you will glow with the relationship that you've encouraged to grow, and be happy because you have made both of them happy.
>
> But days may go by without the benefit of his reading the daily paper! He can be a better person and active citizen of the community if he has a helpful wife who will circle or clip interesting articles to share with him.
>
> A wise man once said: "If your husband invites you to go somewhere with him, go, 'cause otherwise he'll find someone else to take your place!"
>
> [Due to the number of women working in your husband's profession] it becomes apparent that to hold a man you must utilize the same talents as to win a man! The well-groomed, interesting lady who once won his heart must remain!
>
> As the wife of an MD you are looked to for leadership in the community. This is an excellent way for you to develop and gain recognition as an individual, and for your husband to be represented as a part in your achievements.[1]

To most women today, such advice is outdated and insulting. But for some, living such a life is a source of pride and esteem; they *do* embrace the role of junior partner in their husband's life, which revolves around his medical career, and they are proud of this fact.

Here we are not referring only to little old ladies who "just didn't know any better." A 1986 study of newly qualified physicians and their spouses found that physicians' wives, far and away, found gratification in their husbands' career achievements.[2] These and other researchers of physicians' wives have concluded: "It seems that such marriages in the future may work for those women who derive satisfaction from child-rearing and domesticity, do not want a demanding career of their own and do not expect to spend much time with their partner."[3]

Not surprisingly, the husband in such a marriage tends to bask in the position of respect and power that he is assigned, at least initially. The marriage and family revolve around *his* professional demands, *his* emotional needs, *his* fatigue, *his* preferences, and *his* priorities.

Physicians in these traditional marriages enjoy the freedom to fully focus their energies on career pursuits. Also, not surprisingly, these physicians sometimes have difficulty empathizing with the work/family balance issues experienced by colleagues who themselves have career-oriented mates.

Their Hopes

The hope that typically underlies these traditional medical marriages is that, through her infinite love and nurturing, the wife will be able to provide the busy physician with peace and contentment. She expects this, and so does he. Her nurturing presence counterbalances his drivenness and fatigue. Implicit is the expectation that once the husband's quests are attained (education, career success, family, house, and so on), he will relax and join his loving spouse in a more nurturing style of living. These couples clearly embrace the proverbial "psychology of postponement" that already has been discussed.

Their Lifestyle

As the years progress, partners in this pattern often settle into living separate lives. The wife fills her life with activities and friends that stem from her caretaking of children and from other involvements that do not include her husband. Being the stress absorber in the family, she is in charge of praising, pleasing, and cheerleading the family members. Her sense of individuality comes from the friendships and activities that she sandwiches in between caretaking. The reward for this relatively selfless lifestyle is the satisfaction that comes from her being a homemaker and caretaker and the pride that she takes in her family and her husband.

The husband in this pattern, on the other hand, creates an ever-expanding life *outside* his home. In some *We're a Physician* couples, the husband's life fills with increasing variations of a single theme: his own pursuits. Initially, most of them have to do with his role as breadwinner.

He works harder and harder, creating opportunities that he feels compelled to take advantage of, or scrambling to stay afloat in his shark-infested work territory. Eventually, his self-focused style leads to a level of disconnection from his spouse that sets the stage for serious problems in the marriage.

Their Pitfalls

Most often, the initial signs of tension in these traditional medical marriages come in the form of complaints by the wives. Each week in our practice, we see numerous women who are frustrated and depleted in their stress-absorbing roles. They seek our help in dealing with the hurt and anger that stem from their fear that their physician-husbands no longer value the way they run their collective life. We find many variations of dissatisfaction in these marriages.

The "I Need More!" Mistake. As stress and fatigue from excessive career demands accumulate, these physicians often decide that they need a distraction from their lifestyle. With full encouragement (and often prodding) from their nurturing, caretaking wives, many such men then attempt a solution that perpetuates the problem. In trying to gain relief from stress, they try something that exacerbates one of their major stresses.

A classic example of this dilemma is the "If I'm going to work this hard, I'm going to start spending some of this money on stuff that *I* really want" solution. This strategy often leads the stressed medical couple to buy something that requires two things that are already driving them into stress overload: time and money. One of our physician-clients taught us about this creative way of expanding an already overloaded life.

Over the course of last summer, I kept noticing all these patients coming in with perfect tans, telling tales of how much they were enjoying their summer. I was pale and feeling puny; sick and tired of spending my weeks in the office and hospital; even more tired of my weekends doing the same old stuff—nothing much.

So I got this brainstorm, and as usual, I talked my wife into going along. We decided to buy a weekend cottage at Lake Norman. I remember thinking that my on-call schedule was such that, except for every third weekend, we could basically live at the lake summers as long as I was willing to make the easy one-hour commute to my office. I hoped that we could finally start relaxing and connecting as a family. This promised to be a great move!

Of course, in our typical style, we decided that if we were going to use this place, it needed to be nice. To make a long story short, this dream of a little cottage has turned into a $350,000 second-home nightmare.

I don't have the time or interest to maintain my first home, much less this extravaganza complete with a boathouse, decks, and pier that needs to be maintained at the expense of a one-hour drive. I feel more pressure than ever to find time and money. This stress-management plan of mine is about to stress me to death!

The "Getting Serious About Having Fun" Mistake.   Another variation of attempting a solution that perpetuates the problems occurs when an intense, competitive, obsessive physician—again, often with the nurturing encouragement of his spouse—turns to a stress-management ploy that helps soothe his stress but also further isolates him from his wife and family. The solution to one kind of stress simply creates a second stress problem. The classic version of this mistake is taking up a hobby like golf, fishing, or (solo) snow skiing and convincing yourself that attaining true competence is of utmost importance even if doing so requires extended absences from one's family. Remember that, given their tendencies to perceive even hobbies as challenges and to react to challenges with competitiveness, compulsiveness, and perfectionism, any obsessive Type A is at risk of turning a hobby into a *serious* avocation. What starts off as fun and games often ends up stressing rather than soothing. The following comments by Amy about her husband, David, demonstrate this process.

I know and appreciate how hard my husband works. I have never faulted him for this. In fact, I have admired him—almost to the point of holding him in awe. I could never be a physician. I don't know how he manages the pressures that he faces every day. David is a different breed of person from me. He has more high-stakes stress in his life than I do. I am not confused about this.

In fact, I am the one who had to talk him into trying golf. I knew that it would do him good to relax and do something enjoyable with his friends. Otherwise, he just lives in isolation, working himself to death.

My problem is, I don't understand why he has to turn playing golf into such an ordeal and a ritual; his golf has become a major pain in our family's neck. The man is impossible to live with if his Wednesday afternoon or Saturday or Sunday golf games get rained out or preempted by some patient's emergency.

I've got two questions: First, why does he have to play golf so much? If he isn't working, he's on the golf course. Second, why is golf so important to him? He is miserable if he has a bad round, and his life seems to hinge on the outcome of our club's member-guest tournament.

If I do manage to convince him to skip a day of golf in order to do something with me or the kids, he will go along with the plan, but I can tell that he's angry. He pouts, gets irritable, and ruins whatever we are doing with his dour attitude. I feel like I've created a monster.

At first I thought that this was kind of 'cute'—his intensity about a silly game like golf. I teased him about it. But now I don't think that it's so funny. All he cares about is work and golf.

Why Am I Doing This?

It is no surprise that wives in these marriages are at high risk of becoming fatigued, disillusioned, and resentful in response to their husbands' seeming indifference and growing obsession. Further comments from Amy about David's long work hours demonstrate this point.

Oh, he talks a good game: 'I'm doing what I do so that all of us can have a good life' and so on. But the man couldn't tell you the names of his children's schoolteachers if his life depended on it. He doesn't know what our kids' lives are like: what their after-school activities are, when they have exams, or what they worry about.

I'm not saying that I want him as involved in their day-to-day activities as I am; I like the fact that this is my territory. What I am saying is that he doesn't seem to be interested in our life. This is about me and him; this is our life. And—I guess this is the most painful part—he is not interested in me. What am I going to do in five years, when these kids are all grown and gone?

You might argue that we exaggerate with this illustration. If you do, you probably are not living in a *We're a Physician* marriage. Most of the medical wives who reviewed early drafts of this book emphasized that, if anything, we may have softened the picture of such marriages.

As she enters midlife, such a woman confronts haunting self-questioning. She may wonder whether or not she has sold herself out to the allure of this high-powered man who held so much promise of being an affirming partner at the beginning of the relationship, but who now seems to have become self-absorbed and insensitive. She may question whether her nurturing, caretaking style is actually her version of codependent enabling. Maybe if she ran less interference for him, he would be forced to get more involved in the day-to-day details of their personal life. Maybe if she stopped taking up so much of the slack in dealing with their children, he would be forced to be a better parent. Maybe if she gave up being in charge of managing his stress, he would be forced to learn to manage his own.

Where Did the "Good Mother" Go?

When these questions surface, the relationship's contract renegotiation struggle is on. The husband's initial reaction is typically one of loss and longing. He complains, "What ever happened to that all-loving, all-nurturing woman I married?" He also faces his own haunting questions: "Maybe she's changed into someone that I don't really like." "Maybe she's going through some feminine midlife crisis." "Maybe she's clinically depressed." "Maybe she doesn't know how good her life really is." "Maybe she doesn't know how hard it is these days to make the living I make."

Maybe so. But one thing is certain: If either of you is posing such questions—silently or out loud—then it is time to renegotiate the contract that organizes how you perceive each other and how live your life. Otherwise, you run a significant risk of one of several unfortunate outcomes.

The Silent Majority?

The highest risk here is of settling for the most prevalent version of contemporary marriage: a functional relationship of quiet frustration. You lose your passion, intimacy, and eventually your friendship. The other choices are even more dramatic and destructive.

Let's Make *Her* the Patient!

One perverse tendency in marriage is that when we notice that what we are doing is not working very well, we do it harder! Remember, in the *We're a Physician* pattern, the physician-husband is in the power position. Once such a man is confronted with his wife's dissatisfactions, the "doing it harder" dynamic may lead to the physician wielding his most well-honed weapons in dealing with the marital struggle—his medical knowledge and contacts. Diagnosing his wife—and getting cooperation from colleagues in the process—can be an effective way to invalidate *her* feedback that *he* needs to change.

Unfortunately, many wives in these marriages fall prey to such discounting. They fundamentally believe that their stress counts less than their physician-husband's. Many are intimidated by the impression (true or not) that their husband is infinitely more intelligent, important, and entitled than they are. It is difficult to negotiate a more equitable relationship contract with someone when your perceptions and feelings are invalidated and when you feel undeserving of equitable treatment in the first place.

Many years ago, psychiatrist James E. Miles and colleagues wrote of this syndrome and its potentially devastating consequences:

Most frequently it is the wife who presents as the primary psychiatric patient, and it often appears that both the psychiatrist and the physician-husband collude to keep her in that role. The referral is usually from a physician family friend who has become involved at the husband's request. . . . The physician friend becomes aware of the emotional factors existing in the wife presenting with multiple somatic complaints, whom he investigates exhaustively and refers widely without discovering any significant organic basis for her complaints. Or the physician friend is involved in a moment of crisis. . . . Caught between his concern over the wife's condition and his reluctance to label his friend's spouse as a psychiatric patient, the family friend seizes upon the next emotional crisis, often a suicide attempt, to make the psychiatric referral. . . .

Typically, the physician's wife presents as depressed, angry and desperately unhappy. Frequently she is bewildered as to why she is experiencing such feelings. Materially comfortable, with secure social status, usually a financially generous husband, and often envied, her unhappiness and anger may seem inappropriate to her. The husband seems no less bewildered. He has "followed the rules"—worked hard, provided amply and wished the best for his family and is baffled by the turn of events which finds him with a depressed and suicidal wife and problem children. These men tend to be professionally competent and successful, but present as rigid, interpersonally distant and covertly or overtly controlling. They are extremely uncomfortable with feelings, whether of love and tenderness or hostility. They often are successful in demeaning the legitimate and meaningful feelings expressed by their wives by labeling them "emotional outbursts" and making demands for more "logical and rational" methods of problem-solving. Their need to avoid open conflict appears paramount and may, in part explain such phenomena as:

• Prescribing medication for the wife . . .

• Increasing the amount of time spent in the practice, which effectively removes him from the arena of conflict.

• Tolerating the increasingly outrageous behaviors that his angry wife often resorts to as her needs continue to be unmet.[4]

Okay. I'll Be a Patient: In Your Face!

Other struggling *We're a Physician* couples settle into a passive-aggressive dance that revolves around unsolvable medical problems suffered by the seemingly powerless wife. Her unsolvable problem may take various forms: headaches that become chronic, depression that doesn't respond to treatment, fatigue or vague aches and pains that can't be accounted for by any diagnostic findings, or lack of a sex drive despite all efforts on his part to stir her interest. Her problems become a passive form of control in the relationship. He has his foot on the accelerator, but she is applying the weight of her inertia on the brakes in some part of their relationship that is important to him. Guess who has the control, at least in this one area? In this version of triangulation, focusing on the wife's unsolvable problem becomes pivotal in the struggles that originated with the couple's failure to address the problems in their marriage.

Who's Been Sleeping in My Bed?

Less dangerous to one's health but potentially lethal to one's marriage is yet another scenario that often occurs at this juncture in a troubled medical marriage: an extramarital affair. Fortunately, the incidence of extramarital affairs in contemporary marriages is decreasing. But we have found that this *We're a Physician* marital pattern carries particular risks of extramarital involvements for *both* partners.

The physicians in these marriages often harbor a secret: They grow bored with their all-nurturing wives. This boredom makes sense: After all, the women in these relationships tend to blunt the more earthy, zestful, spunky parts of themselves as they fit into the role of maternal caretaker. Even if such a woman tries to integrate her passionate self into her repertoire, her husband may still myopically view her as a "good mother." Accordingly, *he* is likely to discount that *her* passionate self is really an authentic part of her.

The likelihood of entering into a new, exciting, relatively simple and passionate relationship increases for a physician in such a marriage. The physician's increasing self-focus paradoxically combines with a growing sense that, in actuality, he is spending his life taking care of everyone *else's* needs. Self-focused people are typically filled with feelings of anxiety, urgency, and frustration, not with satisfaction from their self-focused behaviors. This frustration boils to a sense of urgency during their midlife reexamination, and their discomfort with family tensions may propel them into a search for another "island of refuge."

Such researchers as Dalma Heyn, author of *The Erotic Silence of the American Wife*, have exploded the myth that only high-powered men are at risk of extramarital affairs. It seems that even the most loving and devoted caretaker-wife is at risk of drifting into an affair if the intimacy in her marriage diminishes.

This research documents a fact that we have observed hundreds of times in our clinical work: Most often, when a woman has an affair, it initially has little to do with sex. When such a woman finds herself giving clear voice to her inner thoughts, needs, feelings, and wants and finds that a high-powered man is once again responding to her in ways that show that he is interested in being a pleasing partner to her, the results are overwhelmingly seductive. She feels *free* to express herself—verbally, emotionally, and eventually, sexually.

This is powerful stuff. The magic that started the romance that once led to the marriage is now fueling an affair that will violate the marriage that has lost its magic.

Pattern 2: The Physician and His Wife: Pleasing Others Even if It Kills Them

Here the caretaker in the medical marriage is a driven Type A woman who is not a physician. In our experience, this is the predominant marital pattern for contemporary high-powered women—both those who are scrambling to combine career and home and those who have sacrificed their own career to focus on managing home and family.

Their Roles

The original relationship contract in this pattern glorifies and romanticizes the woman's high-powered coping style. She is valued as an energetic, no-nonsense person who knows how to manage herself and her life. Most such women are attracted to men who are not threatened by their powerful style, who themselves have a more relaxed style of coping, and who also value their more traditional feminine side. In the course of marriage and family life, such a woman finds unending—and ultimately exhausting—opportunities to show her stamina and skills.

She assumes the role of running the home and of orchestrating a full, enriched, and stimulating life for the family. She is involved in the community or her own professional activities as well as in the lives of her children and spouse.

He is left to focus on medicine and basically assumes a tagalong role in his marriage. His energy goes into his career and into keeping up with whatever his dynamo wife organizes in their personal life. He may make most (or all) of the family's money, but she wields most of the power in the marriage.

Their Hopes

The hopes that underlie this relationship pattern vary, depending on the extent to which the husband is self-absorbed versus nurturing, and on the relative ambitiousness of husband and wife. If the husband has a relaxed, low-key coping style, the relationship starts with the hope that the woman's energy and enthusiasm will add zest to his life. A corresponding hope that often goes unstated is that his measured approach to life will help calm her high-strung coping style. *Her* zest will counterbalance *his* emotional sameness. *His* self-assured peacefulness will help quiet *her* burning ambitiousness or drive to gain social acceptance. In short, his laid-back style is initially framed as quiet strength and maturity.

Yet another important clause in the original relationship contract may go unspoken: The wife is perceived as being in need of the nurturance that was lacking in her first family or in her prior romantic relationships. Basically, the underlying hope is that the husband's love and appreciation will satisfy the wife's need for validation as a person whose value lies not only in achieving, but also in feminine caretaking. She needs a specific form of narcissistic mirroring: gratification of questions regarding her worth as a powerful yet nurturing example of the female species.

At the same time, an ambitious, high-powered woman often enters such a relationship with the unspoken hope that her way of living will become contagious to her mate, and may see him as someone who never really reached his fullest potential. She hopes to help her laid-back partner "discover his own potential." Her hope is that the high-powered lifestyle that she will orchestrate (and that he will modulate) will set a pace and a rhythm that he will learn to enjoy.

If the husband, too, is a driven achiever (as is often the case), then the relationship tends to organize initially around the theme of mutual respect and admiration of each other's power and talents. Both partners recognize the other's high-poweredness and the hope that they will cooperate in constructing an enjoyable, full life. What happens next distinguishes these couples from those who do succeed in this lofty plan (the *Using Our Good Stuff to Make It Better* pattern to be described in Chapter 13).

Their Lifestyle

Regardless of the physician-husband's coping style, these couples tend to settle into a lifestyle that revolves around the female dynamo's activities and reactions. Such women tend to be exceptionally capable and driven. They also crave approval in all that they do, a desire that only grows as the years progress.

A recent survey of 200 academic surgeons and their nonphysician spouses found that 83 percent of the spouses worked in some capacity outside the home, and more than one half of these spouses maintained permanent jobs in addition to assuming responsibility for the rigors of home life. Admittedly, many of these women worked in permanent part-time jobs; only 17 percent of these spouses reported full-time jobs. But, overall, these doctors' wives worked outside their home on average 20.9 hours per week.[5] Much of this effort is in the name of validation, especially in the form of their husband's applause. This fact, coupled with her conflicting needs, may lead such a woman to forgo advancement in her own thriving career in order to satisfy her mate's need for a full-time nurturer. The case study of Beverly and Jim Warren (Chapter 5) was a case in point.

Their Pitfalls

A woman caught in *The Physician and His Wife: Pleasing Others Even if It Kills Them* pattern is at high risk of growing exhausted and depressed as she responds to her need to be all things to all people. And, in the process, she exhausts herself *and* them. Her TYABP magnifies her combination of *Pleasing Others, Being Perfect,* and *Trying Hard* personality drivers (see Chapters 3 and 4). While her steadfast efforts foster many positives, they also may lead to an unexpected double-cross: Irritation by family members may begin to replace the applause.

The physician-husband may struggle to keep up with her energy, pace, and demand for stimulation and excellence. As one physician living in such a marriage lamented: "My life is a piece of cake compared to my wife's. I work hard, but then I relax. She hardly ever stops working. She works at home. She works on the kids. She works the crowd at a party. She works in the Junior League. She works on her body. All the woman ever does is work."

The children in such a family may also resent the wife's drivenness. As the teenage daughter of one such marriage explained to us: "The problem is that my mom is just too intense. She is at every single thing I do. I guess I ought to like that, but I don't appreciate her comments. She wants me to be perfect, like her. She doesn't just tell me that I played or danced well or that I didn't play or dance well. She has to comment on how I looked and how I acted and how I am compared to all of my friends. I know that she loves us, but she drives me crazy."

The shift from applause to criticism of the wife's relentless efforts sets the stage for the couple's contract renegotiation struggles. These struggles can take several forms.

He's Forgotten Who I Am!

If the husband of a *Pleasing Others* Type A female is or becomes very self-absorbed, then both he and she may "forget" who she is. One woman attorney with whom we worked grew depressed from her endless series of disappointing career changes, all made in an effort to find the perfect fit between her career needs and the needs of her physician-husband and two preteen children.

First, with hopes of having more freedom to schedule her office hours around the needs of her children, she resigned her position as a faculty member in a law school and joined a thriving private practice, where she negotiated a reduction in income in exchange for not having to take on trial responsibilities. When even this reduced workload disrupted her family life, she reluctantly took a temporary leave of absence from practicing law.

At last contact, that leave had extended to four years, and this woman was floundering in depression and questioning whether she had made the right decision:

A day doesn't go by that I don't question whether or not I have done the right thing. My parents sacrificed to educate me, and I sacrificed most of my youth to get educated. I was a serious student. During law school, while both of my roommates were smoking grass and listening to Jimi Hendrix, I was in the library, studying.

Now one of those 'wild women' is about to make partner in one of New York's largest firms, and the other is making a fortune running her own practice. And where am I? I'm carpooling.

I'm not saying that I regret the time I'm spending with my children. I cherish them. I even love listening to them banter with their friends when I carpool. It satisfies me on a deep level that I am in their presence as much as I am.

But I'm confused and filled with questions about myself. I feel like I'm losing my confidence. The years are passing, and I am not keeping up with another part of my life that I have always cherished—the law.

If and when I decide to return to practice, I am going to have a lot of catching up to do, and that frightens me. I made it through school, great grades and all, feeling like a fraud. You know, a girl from a blue-collar family knocking them out in the Ivy League. Am I just going through a normal kind of reaction to motherhood? Or, heaven forbid, maybe all of this questioning is because I've lost the little bit of confidence I had in myself as a professional, in the first place.

The worst part of this is that my husband is treating me like I'm a housewife who has no sense. He seems to have forgotten that he is not the only professional in this marriage. I am an attorney who decided to put my career aside for the sake of our family. This was a decision that he and I made together. Problem is, now that his medical career is zooming, he has forgotten who I am; in so many ways, so have I.

Who's the Boss?

The final variation of this pattern tends to be the most problematic. It is a contemporary twist to the traditional medical marriage. Whether or not she is a professional, if a high-powered woman marries a man who does not match her level of ambitiousness and drive, the relationship is likely to settle into a pattern that family therapist Gus Napier identifies as a wife-dominated marriage. Napier claims that these are among the most unhappy of marriages.[6]

Just like male counterparts with similar personality traits, many over-functioning, strong, organized, competent women are also emotionally starved. They yearn to be supported, even though these needs for nurturance may be repressed and redirected into taking care of others.

Like many physicians, women caught in a frenetic *Pleasing Others* style of living typically chart the genesis of this pattern to a childhood that revolved around parental focus on her achievements and caretaking, not on her emotional needs. In fact, Napier notes that, as children, many such women essentially functioned as parents to their own parents or younger siblings. The complementary marital role of such an overfunctioning woman, according to Napier, is the underfunctioning man who both encourages and resents his wife's competence. Often such men enter marriage in search of a strong, caretaking spouse who will soothe the emotional wounds caused by his own rejecting, absent, or ineffectual parents.

One variation of this theme of overfunctioning wife/underfunctioning husband occurs when a high-powered male loses his prestige or employment—an unfortunately frequent scenario in contemporary corporate America. In medical marriages, this pattern of overfunctioning wife/underfunctioning physician-husband more typically leads to struggles over whether or not he will speed up and fit into the Type A wife's way of living. Whether he is indeed underfunctioning or has reached his potential is often a matter of opinion that has serious relationship consequences. Consider the plight of A.J. and Rebecca in the following case example.

A.J. and Rebecca

A.J. always seemed to be moving at half speed, especially in comparison to his dynamo wife, Rebecca. At first, Rebecca viewed A.J. as peaceful and contented with life, and she admired him for his laid-back style. When Rebecca's perspective shifted, relationship struggles flared. She began to see her husband's laid-back style as a symptom of his "chronic lack of ambition." Her irritation grew until she perceived A.J. as "out-and-out irresponsible."

Then came her complaints about A.J.'s "passivity" in running the household and parenting their three children. She also complained about his "lackadaisical" way of managing his medical career.

Next came the role modeling. At the start of every week, she posted his and hers to-do lists on the refrigerator. She redoubled her efforts to appear efficient and responsible. She also began coaching A.J. in ways to make his medium-sized psychiatric practice more successful. She used her own experiences in fundraising and marketing to design ways that her husband might more forcefully market his practice and advance his career.

After years of struggling, Rebecca began to complain of not being interested in A.J. What used to seem calming about him now bored her to tears. The man was content to be less than he could be! Worse, he did not seem interested in "improving himself."

Predictably, A.J., too, began to see his mate in a new and less flattering light. While he used to perceive Rebecca as full of spunk and joie de vivre, he now found her controlling and driven by misplaced values. During one of our counseling sessions he made a clear relationship-renegotiation move as he tried to explain himself to his wife:

"*I know that you have twelve useful points about how I could be more productive around home and work. I know that you see fifteen different ways that I could work more efficiently and expand my practice. I know that you see so much more that I could be.*

"*I also know that you do not understand a very basic point, a point that I have been trying to get across to you for the past five years: Now that I'm all grown up, I know that I do not want to be you. I like myself just as I am. To hear you talk, I'm some sort of slouch around home and a financial and professional failure. The truth is that I make my fair share of contributions in running our home, I am respected by professional peers who matter to me, and I make a very good living.*

"*Now, if you do need for me to change, then we need to have a serious conversation. If you feel dissatisfied with our lifestyle and really want more than we can afford, we need to talk about it. If you need relief from stress or more peace of mind or more companionship, I want to know. But I also need for you to know that it is important to me for you not to decide that I'm a lazy, irresponsible person. I am not. I'm simply not you.*"

Life in the Double Bind

Obviously, the relationship pitfalls for *The Physician and His Wife: Pleasing Others Even if It Kills Them* couples are complex. For the wife, her relentless quest to be and do all leads to a loss of glamour. Without needed appreciation and applause for her heroic efforts, she begins to lose her sense of self. She becomes exhausted and questions the worth of living the lifestyle she has constructed. No matter how great her contributions and effort, she often fears that she has not really achieved enough in any one area of her life. Her bind? If she redoubles her efforts, she grows more exhausted and angry. On the other hand, if she stops trying so hard, she encounters the fears that come to any Type A when faced with a loss of control.

The husband in this marital pattern encounters his own double bind. On the one hand, he might join with his wife in her quest to live out the fundamentally unnurturing script of the driven pleaser. On the other hand, he might resist her pull to become more like her and run the risk of losing her respect.

The Way Out

Renegotiating an overfunctioning/underfunctioning division of roles requires the couple to stretch into unfamiliar territory as individuals and as a couple. Husbands in these marriages must learn to resist passive-aggressive ploys as they struggle with their high-powered mates. Like A.J. in the preceding case example, they must run the risk of clarifying *who* they are and *how* they plan to run their lives while *also* responding compassionately to their mates' valid requests to share responsibilities.

At the same time, wives in these marriages need to learn to share responsibility and power and to validate—not simply criticize—their mates. This means controlling the tendency to project their own conflicts about drivenness onto their partners.

If these issues are not successfully resolved, such couples run the risk of creating a marriage filled with struggle. The wife's relentless quest to be all things to all people exhausts and drains her own and the marriage's vital energy, and the husband's unclear response to the distress in the marriage simply adds fuel to the fire.

References

1. Keil BA. It's not the quantity of time, it's the quality. *J Fla Med Assoc.* 1977;64:105-106.
2. Kelner M, Rosenthal C. Postgraduate medical training, stress, and marriage. *Can J Psychiatry.* 1986;31:22-24.
3. Yandoli AH. Stress and medical marriages. *Stress Med.* 1989;5:213-219.
4. Miles JE, Krell R, Lin T-Y. The doctor's wife: mental illness and marital pattern. *Int J Psychiatry Med.* 1975;6:481-487.
5. Moore EE. Presidential address: swimming with the sharks without the family being eaten alive. *Surgery.* 1990;108:125-138.
6. Napier A. *The Fragile Bond: In Search of an Equal, Intimate and Enduring Marriage.* New York, NY: Harper & Row; 1988.

Chapter 11

Let the Competition Begin!

The most important single factor in the career of a woman doctor is the man she marries—who, I might add, is like anyone else, capable of change.

—Marcia Angell, M.D.,
Deputy Editor, *New England Journal of Medicine*

A 1992 survey found that the vast majority of the female physicians polled were married to men who were in occupations of the same status and that 50 percent were married to other M.D.s.[1] By contrast, contemporary statistics show that male physicians live in households that differ drastically from those of their female colleagues. Only 6 percent of the overall population of male physicians are married to female physicians, and only 20 percent of male M.D.s are married to women of equal professional status. Furthermore, less than 5 percent of male M.D.s are married to women who earn as much money as they do, and only 7 percent have wives who work as many hours per week outside the home as they do.[2,3]

Most often, compared to other women and to male physicians, marriage and family life for contemporary women physicians are especially complex. Marital dynamics have a more pronounced effect on the degree of job involvement for the physician-mother than for a physician-father. Historically, the relationship between family and work involvement was opposite for male and female physicians. If married with kids, male physicians worked more and earned anywhere from 15 to 50 percent more than male M.D.s in other living arrangements. For women physicians, the opposite relationship between family and work occurred: Childless women M.D.s (married or not) earn more money and work somewhat longer hours than their female colleagues who have children. Recent research suggests that, when physicians marry each other, *both* spouses make career sacrifices in deference to family needs. However, the authors of a survey of 1,208 physicians concluded that "in dual-physician families, the professional family lives of both male and female physicians continues to reflect dominant gender roles."[4]

Understandably, the more a woman physician devotes herself to family life and child-rearing, the less her income and career involvement. As we have already mentioned, there are only 168 hours in every week, even for physician-mothers. But another factor may affect the career paths of a woman physician: Like many high-performing women, female physicians may hold back full involvement in their careers in reaction to marital dynamics, not just as a response to time limitations. Even today, when a woman earns more money than her husband, tensions may occur in the marriage.[5] Our glimpses inside the private workings of many medical marriages have led us to believe that this dynamic often plays a significant role in shaping career choices for women physicians.

Of course, many factors account for the discrepancies in female- and male-physician careers, including sexism in medical and academic settings. But our point relates more to personal dynamics (and their marital consequences) than to politics. Why do women physicians often compromise their professional involvements? Portending the aforementioned recent research on dual-physician marriages, University of Chicago family expert Froma Walsh, cofounder of the Chicago Center for Family Health, offered an observation regarding dual-career families that holds for contemporary medical marriages: "Although most mothers are now employed in the workforce, the vast majority of marriage contracts are based on the traditional belief system that a woman's place is in the home."[6]

What Is "Normal" Family Life for Women Physicians?

While women physicians share many of the dilemmas faced by other women in contemporary times, they also face a number of gender-related personal issues that appear to be unique to the stresses and dynamics of their profession. Social researchers Peter Uhlenberg and Teresa Cooney conducted an extensive study of the 1980 US Census data[7] of 1,159 women physicians and 8,820 male physicians and found that at any age more male than female physicians are married. Furthermore, female physicians who do marry tend to do so at an older age. For example, in the age category forty to forty-nine, nearly five times as many female as male physicians never married. At any point along the life span, more female than male physicians are currently divorced. By contrast, females in the United States tend to marry earlier than males, and across the life span, a higher proportion of females than males have ever married.

As will be discussed shortly, the vast majority of women physicians become mothers. However, the fact remains that female physicians are much more likely than their male colleagues to be childless. In the over-forty age category, twice as many female physicians are childless compared to the wives of male physicians.[7]

One thing in our field of study is for certain: Today, more than ever before, fewer families fit the stereotype of the "normal" family—the breadwinner-homemaker model. In fact, experts in the field have questioned whether this stereotype created by the marketing of the 1950s images of *Leave It to Beaver* and *The Donna Reed Show* ever really existed in the privacy of couples' dynamics. For example, Froma Walsh has pointed out that, since preindustrial times, families have always had diverse structures:

> Family disruptions, single parent and remarriage families, and foster and adoptive families were quite common due to the high early mortality rate. The average life expectancy was only 45 years. Families were fortunate— and atypical—if both parents lived to see all their children reach maturity.[8]

We mention this fact in hopes of soothing an ache that we know many physician couples feel. Like many high-powered women, female physicians fear that all that might ail their family is due to their career involvements having taken them "too far afield" from the traditional female role. Even when she *is* doing all of her own domestic work, *is* intimately and lovingly involved with her children (if she has any), and *does* manage to do all of the above and still make more money than most people in the universe, the contemporary woman physician may feel guilty, especially if anyone she loves proves to be like the rest of us and is not blessed with a pain-free life.

More than other people, physicians tend to pathologize. They are trained to interpret symptoms of distress as signs of an underlying illness. In truth, this medical model simply does not always apply to family life. When something is wrong with a loved one or a child, it is not necessarily due to some underlying malady, like one's deficiencies as a parent.

Pattern 3: The Physician and Her Husband: Pleasing Others Even if It Kills Her

What happens when a woman physician marries a nonphysician? If the man is secure, the couple will probably strike a functional bargain. Very likely, the man will be educated, a career-minded professional, and supportive of his wife's medical career—at least at first—but much less support will be typically offered than a nonphysician wife offers a male physician.

Their Roles

Few women enter medical training over the kicking and screaming objections of a resistant husband. Most women physicians (or physicians-to-be) marry men who graciously assume the role of supporter of their wives' medical training or career, respect the women's high-poweredness, and make room in their lives for their wives' grueling training or demanding work. The physician's husband initially takes pride in his role as a liberated, broad-thinking, and supportive man married to a high-powered woman.

A woman physician typically claims her right to pursue her career, negotiating a delay in starting a family and clarifying the limits to which she will be available to assume traditional domestic roles and responsibilities. For many couples, this initial arrangement is complicated when they become parents. Recent data suggests that approximately 85 percent of married women physicians bear children, and that half of physician mothers give birth to their first child during residency.[9] Such women usually appreciate their husbands' liberated, supportive attitude toward having a career-minded wife. In the early years of such a marriage, the husband's merit increases as he stretches beyond the classically socialized male role and defers to his physician-wife's career demands. In fact, he may even interrupt his own career to accommodate her medical training. This last fact markedly distinguishes the marriages of women physicians with non-physician husbands from those who marry fellow M.D.s. In contrast to her women colleagues married to nonphysicians, a woman physician living in a dual-physician marriage is twice as likely as her M.D. husband to interrupt *her* career in deference to his career.[10]

Their Hopes

Our work with women physicians and their nonphysician husbands has left us with concern and compassion for people living with this marital pattern. These couples are often extremely well intentioned but naive about their own underlying hopes, and their blind spots lead them into troubled waters.

Clearly, most such couples enter marriage hoping that the relationship will afford a comfortable balance in life for the female physician. She welcomes a personal life that excludes medicine but expects that the overall balance in her life will allow for her demanding career. Neither the female physician nor her husband assumes that a medical career will be as invasive of their personal life as it is for male physicians and their wives.

Nonphysician-husbands of female physicians tend to be an interesting and diverse lot, especially when it comes to their marital attitudes. Universally, these men are attracted to their wives' high-poweredness. But they clearly harbor a dual hope that portends potholes in the path of the relationship. On the one hand, they hope to be able to validate their mate's feminine aspects. On the other, they hope to derive vicarious esteem from their affiliation with a physician.

Their Lifestyle

In the early stages of a woman physician's career, similar to the experiences of her male colleagues, the benefits of marriage far outweigh the disadvantages. Being married at first helps women physicians manage the stress of their training and early years of practice. Having a husband helps such a woman maintain a sense of constancy in what may otherwise be a disjointed lifestyle.

Many women physicians work part-time after completing training in order to attend to their families. The family's lifestyle then settles into a traditional division of roles as the physician-wife assumes the lion's share of responsibility for running the family and the husband serves as the primary breadwinner. This tends to be a relatively short-lived and somewhat deceptive arrangement. Remember, women physicians, on average, practice twenty-four years of full-time equivalent during the course of their medical careers. Plus, given the extraordinary work demands that are the norm in the medical profession, part-time work for physicians still typically entails working approximately thirty to thirty-five hours per week!

Their Pitfalls

Throughout this book we have stated or implied that in any marriage there is the expectation that to some degree traditional sex roles will be fulfilled. This tends to be the case no matter how politically enlightened a couple might be and regardless of the career status of the spouses. Feminist psychoanalytic writers like Carol Gilligan remind us that females are socialized to base their sense of well-being on connectedness with significant others and participation in nurturant relationships. Men are socialized to value autonomy and achievement. However, this notion is being challenged by contemporary researchers. In fact, both genders appear to derive self-esteem from accomplishments at work, and their emotional states of happiness or depression seem to be obtained from the relationships they have within the family.

But men and women do react emotionally to different forms of support. A recent study published in the American Psychological Association's *Journal of Occupational Health Psychology* found that both family and work hold equal importance for working mothers and working fathers. However, dual-earner fathers reported depression when they perceived lack of spousal support or family role insignificance, whereas dual-earner mothers reported depression if they perceived lack of sharing responsibilities for household tasks.[11]

For the *Physician and Her Husband* couples, two pitfalls can come from the effects of these sorts of dynamics. In most female-physician marriages, the physician's husband who is not an M.D. becomes less supportive of his wife's medical career as the years progress. Some husbands of physician-wives grow to resent their spouses for not ultimately taking up a traditional family role. The complaints of male spouses tend to be the same as those of female spouses in a traditional medical marriage.

Husbands tire of their physician-wives' constant fatigue or unavailability. They begin to resent the fact that the busy physician's career demands preempt the couple's marriage and family life. Similar to wives of male physicians, these husbands resent the slack in family life created by their physician-wives' extended absences from home. They also chafe at the growing conflict over which spouse's career will take priority in dictating the structure of their life.

While the complaints of physicians' husbands who themselves are not physicians sound similar to those of physicians' wives, there is a twist: Physicians' husbands are much more resentful of the demands of medicine than are physicians' wives. It appears that for many men, being supportive and deferential to their wives' career, even at the cost of their own, stretches them too far afield from their socialized sex role.

Not so obvious (but even more prevalent) is the second pitfall. Ostensibly due to the influences of socialization, men and women react differently to excessive work involvement. For men, both self-esteem and a sense of competency are enhanced by increased work involvement. But this is not the case for most career women. Research has shown that, compared to men, women experience a quicker and clearer point of diminishing returns. Beyond a certain point of work involvement, women begin to experience dissatisfaction with their careers *and* threats to their well-being. To a much greater degree, men, on the other hand, tend to experience increased self-esteem and job satisfaction the more involved in their work they become.

A dual disillusionment occurs in many *Physician and Her Husband* marriages: He experiences pronounced ambivalence about her career involvement, and so does she. This struggle—between a female physician and her spouse and between the female physician's career versus domestic needs—can lead to one of several scenarios.

If the physician's husband is less empowered than she either due to his own diminished self-appraisal or to the objective truth that he is less educated or successful, then struggles related to her career can lead to a passive-aggressive quagmire. His resentments become ever more vaguely expressed, fueling her own ambivalence about the competent-physician aspect of herself. Often such couples settle into a subtle form of struggling that erodes mutual respect and marital intimacy.

The comments of Mary Concetta, a pediatrician, about her marriage to Myron, an anthropologist, demonstrate the inner workings of such marriages.

When we got married, Myron's support of me and my career was the envy of every other female resident I knew. He truly was a man who was not threatened by powerful women, and he wore his 'feminine' side so comfortably. He actually seemed to enjoy taking care of me in 'motherly' ways. He packed my lunch or brought me dinner when I was on call. He basically ran our household while I completed my residency. He even chose a nontenure track within his own work so he wouldn't be pressured to do research in the evenings. One of us had to be available to run our personal lives, and he volunteered.

After I was in practice for three years, taking care of other women's babies, I wanted one of my own. Loretta was born during my fifth year out of residency. Myron and I decided that I would cut my practice to half time; it would be his turn to focus more on his career.

So far, does this sound like a medical marriage made in heaven or what? This was supposed to work, right? This is how to 'tag team' it through a dual-career marriage. At least that's what all the books said at the time. What the books didn't say was what happened next.

Myron found out that giving his career the big push did not move it along. The university that he works for revamped his department, and the new chairman would not allow Myron to reenter a tenure track. He also started to complain that, as a nontenured professor, he felt like a second-class citizen. I also think that he just got tired of teaching college students who weren't very interested in learning. His favorite saying became 'I keep getting older and wiser, and they remain young, self-centered, and silly.'

He won't admit this—it's too far removed from his image of himself as a Renaissance man—but I know that he resented the loss of income when I cut back to half-time practice. Plus he felt anxious and worried and pressured to make more money and to become more 'successful.' When he didn't, he stopped acting concerned and started acting angry.

He won't admit that, either. He swears he's not angry, he's just never sexual anymore. He's prone to let comments 'slip out' about the 15 pounds that I have yet to lose since having my baby. He's always tired and preoccupied. He's critical of the way I cook and keep house, and inconvenienced if he has to take care of Loretta on the half days that I have office hours.

It's driving me crazy that he won't talk with me about all of this. I know that he is embarrassed over how typical we have become. He's floundering about his self-worth simply because his career is not as successful as he'd like it to be, just like most men would flounder. That's not who he ever was and not who he likes to be, but that's how he now is.

Just like so many professional women who become mothers, I agonize over how much to work versus stay home. Our financial stress would go away if I just went back to work full-time, but I don't want to miss these years of motherhood. My ambivalence is also complicated by the fact that I love being a pediatrician. I miss my practice. I tried talk-

ing with Myron about my conflict and just ended up crying when I thought of what it would mean to be gone from home as much as I would if I do go back to full-time practice. All Myron had to say was, 'You were the one who wanted to be a physician. Live with it.'

Where did this man come from? This is not who I married. He is not the supportive husband he was during my training. I know that in some ways my going back to work would rub his face in the truth that is hurting him: He is not as financially successful as he might have been if he hadn't made the choices he did to facilitate my career. My own mixed feelings about how much I want to work are bad enough, but his passive-aggressive reactions magnify them by one hundred.

I'm living in a double bind—No! It's a triple bind: I feel damned if I go back to work full-time and have to deal with Myron's anger because I make more money than he does, not to mention my sadness about leaving Loretta. I feel damned if I keep working half-time and have to deal with Myron's anger about our changed lifestyle and my own mixed feelings about taking this break from my career. And I feel damned if I express any of this to Myron and he acts wounded, as though I don't appreciate his dilemma or what he has done in the past to facilitate my career.

Myron's afraid that I'll lose respect for him if he isn't able to take up the financial slack that cutting my practice to half-time has created. I won't. I swear, I won't.

But I will tell you this: I am losing respect for him because of the passive-aggressive way he is taking all of this out on me. I will not stay married to him unless he changes. I guarantee you: I won't put up with being treated like this.

Mary Concetta's ambivalence about her career hints at another factor that complicates the inner workings of female-physician marriages: As women physicians modulate their career involvements in order to focus on child-rearing or other aspects of domestic life, many experience a psychic clash that can be understood by viewing their concepts of self-esteem and competence.

Self-esteem refers to the customary evaluation an individual makes of himself or herself. Am I capable, important, worthy, successful? Self-esteem is generated by successfully handling various facets of life and receiving positive evaluations from others. The result is a global, internalized "I can achieve" attitude. Our experience suggests that few women physicians lack self-esteem. Their string of successes typically results in an internalized sense of worth and capability.

Sense of competence, on the other hand, refers to confidence in one's own abilities to master the tasks that fill one's environment. This is much more targeted. It refers to task-specific confidence, an intrapsychic feeling of confidence that "I am extremely capable at *this* job."

What does this have to do with the plight of women physicians? In our clinical work we have found that, while few women physicians lack self-confidence, many do not possess a sense of competence when it comes to their domestic realm. Simply stated, most of these women, like many of their male-physician colleagues, simply have not spent much time nurturing. Plus, many have had limited romantic experiences and therefore have difficulty ascertaining whether or not their personal life is good enough and, if it isn't, what to do about it. These limitations often lead to haunting, deeply personal questions for these capable women: Am I being a good enough mother? How am I as a lover? Is my husband treating me fairly?

Women physicians who partially, fully, temporarily, or permanently leave their ace-in-the-hole way of promoting both self-confidence and a sense of competence—practicing medicine—need to develop proficiency in an area where they most lack experience. The private dilemma for many such women is that, typically, their husbands view them as all-capable, strong, eminently logical problem solvers—all of the traits that make for a good physician. What both the physician and her husband may have difficulty accepting is her relative insecurity when it comes to the domestic realm. For many women physicians, like Maria in the following case study, these uncomfortable feelings may surface when dealing with women whose sense of competence primarily revolves around that which the female physician lacks.

Maria, a surgeon and the mother of two children aged five and nine, came to the office for the treatment of depression. Since the birth of her youngest child, she had cut her practice by 75 percent in order to be involved in her family life. Her depression began during the third year of her transition from full-time to part-time medical practice. In the following passage she describes a private aspect of her discontent.

Okay. You told me to think about this; to notice during the past week when I feel sad or bothered and what is going on when those feelings occur. I told you I had no idea what this was all about. I lied. I knew one thing as soon as you asked, and I've noticed it even more during this week. I lied because I'm embarrassed about this. And I'm also angry that it's true.

For the first time in my life, I spend a fair amount of time hanging out with other women who are not career women. I take my children to play with their friends, and I have to deal with 'the mothers.' At the pool there are 'the mothers.' At my son's ball games, 'the mothers.' I am uncomfortable around these women, with their perfectly manicured nails, slim-and-trim behinds, and endless chitchat. I used to be oh so comfortable letting it stop there. 'These women are sort of silly. I've got important things to do, so I must go—in a hurry! 'Bye!'

Well, now I don't go; I stay. And what I find is that these women stir more than just criticism in me. Some of what I feel is envy. These women are so comfortable in their totally feminine role. They seem so comfortable chitchatting with each other and keeping up with all of those motherly things, half of which drive me crazy. I know I'm doing this mother thing well enough. But I just don't seem to be as comfortable with all of this as I should be.

There's another part of what happens inside me when I'm around 'the mothers.' I feel left out. This is painful for me to talk about. I was always smarter than most girls I knew throughout school; at least I made better grades than they did. But I was never very popular. It's just a fact. It's not that I want to be best friends with the other mothers; it's just that this feeling of being on the outside of the circle brings back some old-time discomfort that I no longer can soothe in the same old way—by going to work.

So that's that. Another place that I've noticed feeling sad is at home, when I'm alone with my children. I love these children. I love holding them and talking with them and helping them and playing with them. But motherhood leaves me feeling less comfortable and confident than I am accustomed to feeling. I don't really enjoy running my household. It's not definitive enough. I'm used to diagnosing the problem, solving it, or removing it and then sewing the patient up and moving on to the next problem. Obviously, I'm struggling with a part of motherhood and womanhood that I'm not very familiar with.

Just to complete the picture of myself as the mess that I am becoming, now that I'm doing less surgery, I feel like I'm losing my place as 'one of the boys' in the operating room. I'm afraid that I'm going to lose my touch. I love doing surgery. I want to do lots of surgery, and I know that if I don't, I will lose my skills.

So I've done my psychotherapy 'homework.' I now know in vivid detail how, when, and where I feel miserable. What's next?

Whether they are comfortable with their more "feminine" side and whether they work full- or part-time in medicine, there is no doubt that women physicians struggle with inner conflict about multiple roles and that they tend to fill their lives with efforts to come to some balance in those roles. Unfortunately, this effort often results in a variation of the *Pleasing Others Even if It Kills Them* pattern discussed in the preceding chapter, this time with the additional burden of the stresses that come with being a physician. It has been proposed that the well-documented propensity of married female physicians to suffer from periods of depression and an overriding sense of futility may come from the demands of serving as caretaker for patients and as primary caretaker of the emotional needs of her family. Both the physician and her husband may come home at the end of a busy day feeling depleted. But while he feels satisfied by another day of hard work, *she* feels guilty that she has so little energy left to nurture her family. The result is a depression-generating lifestyle that preempts any time or energy for the married female physician to focus on that all-important arena of *self:* She doesn't exercise, play, relax, or even get enough sleep.

By shrinking the "attending to self" factor, these female physicians can jam every other task into 168 hours per week. Studies[12-15] of the combined at-home and at-office work habits of contemporary professional women have consistently shown that normally they work eighty-six to 107 hours a week, even when they do not have children living at home. Further, it appears that, at least in some senses, their overall stress load increases once a husband enters the picture. For example, a recent survey of 581 men and 608 women, married and unmarried, found that married women performed fourteen hours more housework each week than single women. This study also noted men's tendency to overestimate their own involvement in housework and to underestimate how much time other family members spend on it.[15] And a survey of eighty-seven women physicians in Detroit found that three fourths of the women actually did all of their own domestic work: the cooking, shopping, money management for the household, and taking care of the children. Even if they did not perform the tasks themselves, virtually all of them accepted full responsibility for seeing that their household tasks got done by somebody.[16]

Why would an intelligent, empowered, resourceful, educated, sophisticated woman living in the 1990s treat herself this way? Our prior comments regarding research on maternal gatekeeping may apply here. However, we believe that a major part of what fuels this process is institutional and societal intolerance of any alternative. Gender expert Joseph Pleck pointed out that the traditional gender-role norms allow men's work roles to intrude on their family roles but not the reverse. Women's family roles are permitted to intrude on their work roles but not the reverse.[17]

While this statement applies to many professional women, it is only partly applicable to women physicians. In truth, women physicians' family roles are *not* permitted to intrude on their work roles. For example, despite the fact that 63 percent of pregnancies during graduate medical training are planned, as recently as 1989, only 47.8 percent of 366 training hospitals surveyed granted formal maternity leave.[18] This figure has improved: now, more than 75 percent of residency programs report standard maternity leave policies.[19] However, the picture is more bleak post-training. In a 1992 survey of 475 female physicians not in solo practice who were surveyed post-medical training, only one third stated they worked in settings that had a maternity leave policy.[20] And the notion of paternity leave remains virtually unreported in the medical literature.

Reactions of peers and superiors to pregnancy tend to be critical and can be detrimental to a woman physician's career. Following a sanctioned pregnancy leave, women physicians have reported being victimized by an unspoken rule: "you lose out in the 'good ol' boy' system if you don't act like one of the boys." Upon returning from pregnancy leave, women physicians have reported various obvious and subtle forms of peer rejection, including being passed over for committee assignments and other career activities and being the target of open scorn and criticism.

Perhaps these gut-wrenching conflicts contribute to the relatively high rate of emotional distress in women physicians. Many report feeling that they have done much in their lives (established a profession, created a family, and so on) but have not done any one thing very well.

Our claim that the *Physician and Her Husband* pattern, even when it works, revolves around ambivalence about the wife's career is supported by Canadian researchers who polled 200 women physicians and their husbands.[21] The researchers posed the question, "Would you have any advice for young men considering marrying a woman physician?" The husbands' response could be summarized in this way: "Think twice—then go ahead." Advice from the couples in this study included:

- Have good household help.
- Remember to honor the physician-wife's profession: Accept it and show pride in it.
- If possible, wait to have children until *after* the rigors of medical training are completed.
- Remember to communicate.

Pattern 4: Ready, Set, Go! The Physicians and Other Dual-Career Couples

Most often, when two physicians (or a physician and a fellow professional) marry, they create a life that seems like a race. We call this the *Ready, Set, Go!* pattern. The hallmark of this pattern is competition between the spouses that leads to struggles as their collective drive, energy, and talent propel them to constantly expand their life, but prohibits either partner from functioning as a stress absorber in the marriage.

Their Roles

Here the spouses are initially attracted to each other's high-powered, high-energy zest for life. They believe they have found in each other a mirror image, someone who will share their passion for medicine and cooperate in their quest to gain it all—a fast-paced lifestyle, financial success, perhaps a family filled with high achievers, and fun and stimulation along the way. They believe they have finally found a "companion partner," someone who will inherently understand the joys and struggles of a life in medicine and who will, through all the years to come, facilitate satisfaction of the other's strong need for stimulation. Accordingly, they assume that each will constantly give 100 percent effort and remain stress-hardy as they create and manage an ever-expanding lifestyle.

Their Hopes

Researchers of dual-physician marriages claim that with amazing frequency the underlying hope in these relationships is that the more traditional sex roles will eventually evolve.[4,22-23] Once all the trappings of the perfect life are attained, he will end up the primary wage earner, while she will have the option of giving more clear-cut expression to her feminine side with his applause and admiration for her power and capability as an independent person.

Writing of their experiences in counseling dual-physician couples, Case Western Reserve professors of psychiatry R. Taylor Segraves and Kathleen Segraves described this dynamic:

> The marriage may be considered a partnership of equal companions. This may, however, be largely illusion. In fact, both partners may have assumed a more traditional stance, that of a superior, strong male and a more helpless, dependent female. . . . Once the woman advances in her profession and challenges these traditional roles, problems begin to emerge in the marriage.[24]

We fully realize the potential heresy in the above paragraph, particularly for many female physicians. We are *not* implying that we find women physicians to be any less serious about their careers than are their male counterparts. We are certainly not implying that women are any less capable as professionals. We are simply reflecting what we believe to be the very valid observations of such contemporary female writers as Betty Friedan *(The Second Stage)*, Clarissa Pinkola Estes *(Women Who Run With the Wolves)*, Sarah Ban Breathnach *(Simple Abundance)*, and Christiane Northrup *(Women's Bodies; Women's Wisdom)*, who remind us that wholeness for the contemporary woman involves both claiming the right to give full and unencumbered expression to more "masculine" operational aspects of herself *and* incorporating into her life the unique richness of more traditional "feminine" roles and inclinations.

This does not mean that every high-powered woman will ultimately forgo her career in order to become a housewife or grandmother (even though some women professionals we know have done exactly that). This *does* mean that high-powered dual-physician couples will inevitably face a period of contract renegotiation that revolves around the theme of one or both of them wanting a taste of traditional relationship process. Sam Osherson, writing of the dilemmas faced by contemporary men, notes: "Today, many men work hard, but they may not feel like they've gotten the girl, because the girl is also working hard and not able to focus her attention on him in the ways he expected."[25] As we will discuss below, it is also true that today many women work hard, but they may not feel they've gotten their due because the man is so busy with his own quests that he is not able to focus his attention on her in the ways *she* expected.

Their Lifestyle

Due either to their demanding work schedules or to geographic separations that may come with completing training, many dual-physician couples endure periods of long-distance or commuter marriage: Two households are set up in different locations, and the couple reunites when schedules permit. In this way, work and family lives are compartmentalized. During days away from home, each is totally involved in work, with no interference from family demands. When reunited, the couple's time and attention are focused on the family and on household tasks.

A growing number of couples are choosing this unconventional solution to the dilemmas that come with dual careers. No definitive data are available regarding how prevalent this arrangement is in medical marriages, despite claims that this pattern is becoming commonplace during the training period for dual-physician couples. It is generally estimated that in the U.S. population alone there are over one million commuter marriages. This pattern works best for couples who don't have to work on weekends—an obvious problem for most physicians, especially those in training.

As stated earlier, the man's medical career typically takes priority over that of the wife-physician. Many women physicians prefer a less ambitious career course than their husbands and are willing to make the sacrifices needed in order to promote their husbands' careers. However, such women physicians seldom realize exactly what they have bargained for in terms of the overall responsibility that they end up with after the "negotiating" is done. Other women end up deferring to their husbands' careers out of coercion, not choice.

This last statement hints at an often overlooked point: It is important to be sensitive not only to the crucial issue of what effect a woman physician's career has on her family life, but also what impact her family has on the woman physician's career. It has repeatedly been shown that the primary determinant of career involvement for a female physician is her level of responsibility for home and hearth. The formula here is not surprising: The more home responsibilities she has, the fewer hours per week she will work in medicine.

Recent studies of dual-physician marriages have shown that, during training, these couples usually work out a very egalitarian arrangement for dividing home responsibilities. However, once training is completed, a more traditional division of labor is adopted in the vast majority of dual-physician marriages. Specifically, studies of dual-physician marriages suggest that more than 76 percent of women physicians do all the cooking, shopping, child care, and money management for their families. In contrast, only 40 to 60 percent of women physicians married to nonphysicians assume primary responsibility for any single domestic task.[10]

In this sense, dual-M.D. marriages are no different from other dual-career marriages. In dual-career families, employed wives continue to assume more than 80 percent of household and child-care responsibilities, including the overall coordination of family life.[26] This statement is supported by a recent survey of nearly 3,000 randomly selected men and women.[27] Even in the postfeminist United States, women are still two times more likely to pay household bills than men, five times more likely to cook for the family, five times more likely to do the family shopping, and eleven times more likely to do the household cleaning. Most remarkable is that these findings were true even for young couples in which the women contributed half or more of the family income.

As we stated earlier, to truly understand the inner workings of dual-M.D. marriages, it is necessary to recognize another fact: The majority of women physicians today, including those in dual-physician marriages, are highly productive members of their profession in *addition* to running their homes. A study conducted at Johns Hopkins University surveyed 1,420 active obstetrician-gynecologists,[28] over half of whom were women trained during the 1970s. The women in this study were on the average thirty-four years old. The responses of these contemporary, postfeminist-era women physicians indicated that, on average, they worked in medicine 7.5 fewer hours per week than their married male-physician counterparts. However, they still worked, on average, over sixty hours per week and contributed over 50 percent of the total paid work time in their marriages. A 1999 study of 1,208 physicians[4] found that, regardless of the profession of their husbands (i.e., physician or nonphysician), women physicians work forty-two to forty-nine hours per week outside the home, despite the fact that the majority of these women physicians made career sacrifices in deference to their families' needs.

Clearly, having responsibility for running their families shapes career choices for many women physicians. It is a well-known fact that female physicians gravitate toward nonsolo-practice settings: This is not due to lessened time demands in such work settings. In fact, institution-based practice or group practice affiliations typically lead to more, not fewer, numbers of hours spent at work. The crucial benefit that working in these settings offers is greater predictability of work schedules—a *must* for any person charged with child rearing, carpooling, home management, and so on.

Their Pitfalls

Dual-physician couples living the *Ready, Set, Go!* pattern run the risk of stumbling on the by-product of their driven lifestyle: Their competitiveness, diminished intimacy, and lack of a stress absorber in the system, coupled with their longing for more simplicity in their personal life, lead to a growing resentment of the lives they have created.

In the *Ready, Set, Go!* pattern (as in the Superperson state discussed in Chapter 4), a physician may be unaware of his or her own increasing physical or mental fatigue. This process has been poignantly described in studies of role conflict in female university faculty members. Despite working between eighty-six and 107 hours per week in the office and at home, such women tend to consider themselves *not* overworked! As one researcher put it:

> Not only did they not acknowledge that they were overworked, they also took for granted that they ought to be able to accept their dual role without complaint. In not admitting they were overworked, these women felt they could and should be able to be feminine, successful in their careers, good mothers, and have happy marriages—all without feeling overloaded. Taken together, these results suggest that professional women with children living at home appear to have very high standards about combining career and family.[29]

Living in this sort of frenetic activity has negative consequences on a dual-physician marriage. Such couples find it difficult to maintain enough connection to remain intimate. All measures of intimacy may dwindle—how frequently they make love, how often they express nonsexual physical affection, how often they remember the last conversation they had, how often they say nice things to or about each other.

As their lives fill with responsibilities and activities, their relationship may begin to seem like a suffering contest complete with comparisons of who has the busiest schedule today, the most pressured week, or the worst headache tonight. As your collective exhaustion drains their time and energy for romance, the *Ready, Set, Go!* couple may become a "TINS" (two incomes, no sex) couple.

We again emphasize that this pattern is worst during times when both physicians are working full-time. We have known, however, a number of dual-physician couples who were living temporarily on one income in which the at-home mate (in our experience, this has always been the wife) was even more caught up in a time-urgent, stress-generating style of living than was the partner who was still practicing medicine. In such instances, the effect on marital intimacy is the same as if both physicians are working full-time: Neither has the time, energy, or inclination to nurture the other, and pitfalls in the relationship accumulate.

The following two case vignettes exemplify this process.

Elizabeth and Jim

Elizabeth was a full professor of internal medicine at a prestigious medical school. She was internationally known for her research in gastrointestinal disorders. Her abilities and successes were a source of pride and esteem for her husband, Jim, a dermatologist in private practice. In their early years of marriage this couple negotiated a very realistic and respectful contract that was truly egalitarian. For many years Elizabeth and Jim enjoyed a smoothly functioning, caring relationship.

It was a surprise to Elizabeth when she began to lose romantic interest in her husband and feel attracted to other men. It was a shock to her—and, at first, rather insulting to Elizabeth's feminist beliefs—when she finally noticed a common theme in these attractions: The men seemed powerful and traditional in their treatment of women but, at the same time, weren't threatened or sexist in their response to high-powered females.

Elizabeth eventually decided that what she yearned for was a bout of traditional romance. As she expressed it: "I know that I have a right to my career and to my share of independence. I know that Jim is respectful of this fact. He and I harbor no illusions about sex roles or expectations within our marriage.

"But I want more than equality in my marriage. I want some romance! I want a man to 'touch my heart' in some of those old-fashioned male-female ways! I want a man to open doors for me, write poetry to me, and give me romantic surprises—with no illusions of controlling me.

"I was talking about this with my friend, who is also the woman who is my housecleaner. She seems so clear about who she is: a mother, a wife, a woman having an affair with a passionate lover, and a housecleaner. After she listened to me go through all my existential rumblings, she summed it up quite nicely: 'Sounds like you are just now figuring out that a little bit of macho ain't bad.'"

Mitch and Julia

Mitch had no confusion about the relative importance of his and his wife's medical careers. His own cardiology practice was thriving. Julia was the managing partner in an emergency medicine group and served as medical director for a large pharmaceutical research company. She also traveled internationally, speaking at pharmaceutical and medical

meetings. Mitch enjoyed the financial security that came from Julia's suc-
cess, and he admired and respected her combined clinical and research
talents.

Mitch's growing resentment of his wife did not have to do with any
discounting of her power, prestige, or rights in their marriage. He simply
had grown tired of their constantly having to negotiate the caretaking of
their two teenaged children and the management of their home. He came
to counseling on the insistence of Julia, who had grown tired of his sar-
castic comments and sullen withdrawal from her.

Mitch explained his dilemma in these words: "I don't know what is
going on with me. I know that if I were married to some passive, depen-
dent woman, it would drive me crazy. I would never be faithful to such a
woman; I wouldn't stay in such a marriage. I am attracted to high-ener-
gy, independent women.

"But I swear, I get tired of Julia's big life. Every week, she is busier
and more stressed than I am. The most urgent drama in our life each
week is figuring out the flow chart that specifies which of us will be
available to attend our kids' activities, take care of household chores,
and otherwise manage our personal life. I get tired of her constantly
being late when it is her turn to carpool the kids, of her always being in
such a rush, of her never relaxing.

"I'm tired of her having two careers. Sometimes I just wish that she
would carve out a smaller life: declare herself what she is—the senior
partner in a multimillion-dollar practice—and start being more selective
about her research projects.

"We used to have this private joke. We'd look around our messy
house, exhausted from another big day. After sitting there for a while, try-
ing to decide which version of take-out food we were going to eat that
night or whose turn it was to put the kids to bed, Julia would smile and
say, 'What we need around here is a good wife; I wish we could hire one.'
We'd both laugh. The problem is, I don't find it so funny anymore."

It seems inevitable that dual-physician marriages eventually fill with
laments from one partner or both that they need help slowing down,
shrinking the size of their life together, and learning to enjoy the here and
now. The fundamental problem is that usually neither person believes any
renegotiation of their lifestyle is possible. They fear their partner's sabotage of any effort to "slow down," a fear that often masks their own
ambivalence about the warring parts of themselves that want both a nurturing life and high levels of action.

A final pitfall in the path of many such couples harks back to the
aforementioned warning by Segraves and Segraves: what happens in a
dual-physician marriage when the traditional dynamic of strong
male–dependent female is disrupted by a woman physician's coming of

age? As we noted in Chapter 3's discussion of personality development, the balance in a marriage can be seriously tipped by new layers of personality that emerge with maturity, especially if the other partner refuses to change in harmony.

How does this process apply to *Ready, Set, Go!* physician marriages? According to Segraves and Segraves, as the female physician comes of age, she stops idealizing her husband and starts viewing him more as an equal.[24] This shift, in turn, affects the husband-physician's perceived status within the marriage, and struggle ensues. The struggle often involves discounting the validity of the wife's changes, a pattern that was described in the case study of Edie and Simon. "Thus one partner may not accept the other as an independent, competent professional. Worse still, the spouse may act as if the partner has not changed at all during the years of professional development."[24]

We have known dual-physician couples who resorted to unfortunate measures in an effort to stop the conflict that comes with this type of power imbalance. In cases like this, to reinstitute the male-in-power balance that was part of their original contract, the accomplished wife-physician returns to the one-down position in the relationship by developing a problem—substance abuse, an eating disorder, an affective disorder, inability to manage the stress of family life, or disillusionment with her profession. Even though she may no longer need her husband's help facing the challenges of becoming an accomplished physician, by putting herself one-down, she keeps him in the familiar position of one-up to her at the expense of her own well-being.

A marriage cannot grow unless both partners have accurate, up-to-date perceptions of themselves and each other. The fundamental problem faced by couples caught up in the *Ready, Set, Go!* pattern is that they don't slow down enough to *notice* whom they are married to *now*. The constant flurry of action that fills these marriages is what psychiatrist Perry Ottenberg described many years ago as a version of "neurotic health" evidenced by many physicians.[30] Fueled by their quests for perfection, many physicians develop a lifestyle that is characterized by three factors:

- Denial of any symptoms
- Ego investment in achieving success and defining "successful" as not having any problems
- Defining health in terms of having freedom and a balanced life, even if a frenetic pace of activities is necessary to create all of the above.

Dual-physician couples would do well to heed Ottenberg's counsel: "Frenetic activity, no matter how 'balanced,' is not the prescription for emotional health."[30]

The Positive Side of Life in a Dual-Physician Marriage

Despite potential pitfalls, dual-physician couples do have a tremendous potential advantage over all other medical-marriage patterns: the opportunity to show to each other true understanding and compassion about the stresses that come from trying to combine medicine, marriage, and family life. By definition, dual-M.D. couples share many characteristics that aid compatibility. Similarities of training and work experiences can heighten empathy and tolerance of the stresses of the profession. And when both spouses are physicians, it is often easier to feel connected as they share in each other's joys and passion about medicine.

A recently published study of dual-physician marriages suggested that many dual-physician couples benefit from their similarities.[31] A survey of twenty-one such couples showed them to be sympathetic partners who were supportive of each other's careers, good communicators, and reasonably satisfied with their sex lives. These couples rated their marriages high and expressed their mutual appreciation of the understanding shown by both partners of all aspects of being a physician.

The authors of this study offered several points of advice for dual-physician couples that are worth underscoring:

- One spouse's career must take precedence, and a decision should be made in advance about to whose career that should be.
- Decide in advance whether to have children during training or after (if at all).
- Compromise, communicate, and discuss priorities.
- Have realistic expectations about your career and family balance.
- Plan ahead.
- Do not let your interests become too narrow.

We would add here the most crucial key to keeping a medical marriage alive: When the going gets rough, renegotiate!

References

1. Gross EB. Gender differences in physician stress. *JAMA*. 1992;47:107-114.
2. Lorber J. *Women Physicians: Career, Status and Power*. New York, NY: Tavistock Publications; 1984.
3. Uhlendberg P, Cooney TM. Male and female physicians: family and career comparisons. *Soc Sci Med*. 1990;30:373-378.
4. Soebecks NW, Justice AC, Hinze S, et al. When doctors marry doctors: a survey exploring the professional and family lives of young physicians. *Ann Intern Med*. 1999;130:312-319.
5. Sotile WM, Sotile MO. *Beat Stress Together: The BEST Way to a Passionate Marriage, a Healthy Family, and a Productive Life*. New York, NY: John Wiley & Sons; 1999.

6. Walsh F. Meeting the challenges of "normal" families. *Fam Ther News.* 1992;23:7-22.
7. Uhlenberg P, Cooney TM. Male and female physicians: family and career comparisons. *Soc Sci Med.* 1990;30:373-378.
8. Walsh F, McGoldrick M, eds. *Living Beyond Loss: Death in the Family.* New York, NY: Norton; 1991. Cited in: Walsh F. Meeting the challenges of "normal" families. *Fam Ther News.* 1992;23:7.
9. Stephen PJ. Career patterns of women medical graduates 1974-1984. *Med Educ.* 1987;21:255-259.
10. Tesch BJ, Osborne J, Simpson D, Murray SF, Spiro J. Women physicians in dual-physician relationships compared with those in other dual-career relationships. *Acad Med.* 1992;67:542-544.
11. Schwartzberg N, Dytell RS. Dual-earner families: the importance of work stress and family stress for psychological well-being. *J Occup Health Psychol.* 1999;1:211-223.
12. Greenglass ER. Type A behavior, career aspirations, and role conflict in professional women. In: Strube MJ, ed. Type A behavior. *J Soc Behav Pers.* 1990;5(special issue):307-322.
13. Yogev S. Are professional women overworked? Objective versus subjective perception of role loads. *J Occup Psychol.* 1982;55:165-169.
14. Hochschild A. *The Second Shift.* New York, NY: Avon Books; 1990.
15. Bird CE. Gender, household labor, and psychological distress: the impact of the amount and division of housework. *J Health Soc Behav.* 1999;40:32-45.
16. Heins M, Smock S, Jacobs J, et al. Productivity of women physicians. *JAMA.* 1976;236:1961-1964.
17. Pleck JH. Paternal involvement: levels, sources, and consequences. In: Lamb ME, ed. *The Role of the Father in Child Development* (3rd ed.). New York, NY: Wiley; 1997:66-103.
18. Council of Teaching Hospitals. *Cost Survey of House Staff Stipends, Benefits and Funding.* Washington, DC: Association of American Medical Colleges; 1989.
19. Resident Forum. AMA-RPS instrumental in achieving new maternity leave policy. *JAMA.* 1991;265:1756.
20. Baker NJ. Maternity leave for practicing family physicians. *J Fam Pract.* 1992;35:39-42.
21. Vincent MO, Hill MM, Tatham MR. The physician's marriage, husband, family and practice. *Ontario Med Rev.* July 1976:350-356.
22. Sotile WM, Sotile MO. Today's medical marriage: part 1. *JAMA.* 1997;277:1180c.
23. Sotile WM, Sotile MO. Today's medical marriage: part 2. *JAMA.* 1997;277:1322.
24. Segraves K, Segraves RT. When the physician's marriage is in trouble. *Med Aspects Hum Sexuality.* 1987. p 153.
25. Osherson S. *Wrestling With Love: How Men Struggle With Intimacy, With Women, Children, Parents, and Each Other.* New York, NY: Fawcett Columbine; 1992:171.
26. McGoldrick M, Anderson C, Walsh F. *Women in Families.* New York, NY: Norton; 1989. Cited in: Walsh F. Meeting the challenges of "normal" families. *Fam Ther News.* 1992;23:7.
27. Study conducted by the Family and Work Institute, as reported in: Taffel R. The power of two. *Fam Ther Networker.* September/October 1994:44-55.

28. Weisman CS, Teitelbaum MA. The work-family role system and physician productivity. *J Health Soc Behav.* 1987;28:247-257.

29. Greenglass ER. Type A behavior, career aspirations, and role conflict in professional women. In: Strube MJ, ed. Type A behavior. *J Soc Behav Pers.* 1990;5(special issue):319.

30. Ottenberg P. The physician's disease: success and work addiction. *Psychiatr Opin.* 1975;12:6-11.

31. Johnson CA, Johnson BE, Liese BS. Dual-doctor marriages: career development. *Fam Med.* 1992;24:205-208.

Further Reading

For further information on maternity leave during medical training:

AMA Ad Hoc Committee on Women Physicians. *Maternity Leave for Residents.* Chicago, Ill: American Medical Association; 1984:1-21.

Eskenazi L, Weston J. The pregnant plastic surgical resident: results of a survey of women plastic surgeons and plastic surgery residency directors. *Plast Reconstr Surg.* 1995;95:330-335.

Young-Shumate L, Kramer T. Pregnancy during graduate medical training. *Acad Med.* 1993;68:792.

Resident Forum. AMA-RPS instrumental in achieving new maternity leave policy. *JAMA.* 1991;265:1756.

Rile CA, Jagiella V, Michaeletz-Onody P, et al. Parental leave for trainees in gastroenterology: position paper—American College of Gastroenterology. *Am J Gastroenterol.* 1992;87:1358-1371.

For information on maternity leave post-medical training:

Baker NJ. Maternity leave for practicing family physicians. *J Fam Pract.* 1992;35:39-42.

Chapter 12

The Strugglers

Oh! It is excellent to have a giant's strength; but it is tyrannous to use it like a giant.

—William Shakespeare, *Measure for Measure*

Each of the patterns of medical marriage described thus far is complex and stress-filled. However, none can compete with the levels of marital strain and emotional wear and tear that come with the next two patterns. Though quite different in appearance, both revolve around a common theme: remaining stuck in one of the Type A triad of states that were discussed in Chapter 2—Superperson, Depression, and Anger.

Pattern 5: Chaotic Desperation: When Hot Reactors Kill the Love

The *Random House Dictionary of the English Language* (second edition) defines the term "chaotic" as "completely confused or disordered." Any relationship that revolves around the emotional, behavioral, and physiological reactions of a hot reactor can be described with this one word.

In the professional literature, the term *hot reactor* typically refers to any individual who responds to stress with elevated blood pressure and hormonal changes. We use the phrase to describe someone who experiences extreme physical, behavioral, and emotional reactions to stress. These are the people who experience psychophysiological "spinouts" when frustrated, especially when dealing with relationship conflict. They experience such a bath of stress hormones that it is tremendously difficult for them to control their behavior or emotions during a stressful event or to calm down once it is over. They react to stress with excessive anger, blame, or even rage.

Either or both partners in the *Chaotic Desperation* pattern may be a hot reactor. We have seen many high-powered people progress from garden variety TYABP to hot reactivity as the stresses and demands of their lives escalated. For most, however, signs of hot reactivity were there from the start of the relationship but were ignored during the bliss of infatuation. This pattern is likely to occur in people who combine excessive needs for control, hot tempers, and TYABP tendencies *with* the stresses of an overwhelming life.

Their Roles

Regardless of the sex of the hot reactor or whether one or both partners are hot reactors, the original relationship contract in *Chaotic Desperation* marriages tends to be a promise that the *other* spouse's nurturing and tolerance will keep the hot reactions from getting out of hand. This same love and nurturing will allow the hot reactor to recover from his or her need to battle with the world; the nurturing spouse will run interference in order to make the hot reactor's life easier. The spouse implicitly agrees to be all that is different from the hot reactor's impatient, sometimes violent way of reacting to stress.

If the hot reactor's mate is naturally calm and patient, the contract makes sense. After all, that partner's calm style suits the hot reactor's need for a soothing influence. Such partners often hope the hot reactor will add spice, zest, and power to their own lives. The hot reactor is attracted to the partner's peacefulness. The "peaceful" partner is attracted to the hot reactor's energy and forthright manner. At the contracting stage of the relationship, they both assume that the calming influence of the marriage will eventually soothe these temper outbursts away.

A puzzling aspect of many *Chaotic Desperation* relationships is that *both* partners may be hot reactors, but even so, the same initial contract organizes the marriage. It might seem peculiar that a hot reactor who has difficulty calming himself or herself would enter into a contract that specifies that he or she will be a source of calming for the other person. But remember: relationship contracts are most often based on selective perceptions and wish-fulfilling fantasies, not on realistic appraisals of the two partners involved.

Their Hopes

For a hot reactor, the hope underlying the relationship is: "I have finally found a place where I will be tolerated and loved despite myself." The spouse's underlying hope is: "With enough love and support, my partner will grow up enough to act decently." If the spouse, too, is a hot reactor, an additional hope lurks beneath the relationship contract: "Maybe by helping the other person calm down, I will finally gain more control over my own emotional outbursts. If I can help my partner learn to do this, I'll learn to do it, too."

Their Lifestyle

Couples in this pattern soon settle into just what was contracted for: The "calm" partner runs interference, trying to smooth the hot reactor's path, and the hot reactor struggles in his or her attempts at self-control. The household is organized in an attempt to keep the hot reactor calm. If they have children, the calm partner coaches them to behave so as not to annoy the hot reactor. The spouse and other family members generally walk on eggshells in hopes of preventing yet another emotional outburst.

Of course, no amount of vigilance proves effective all of the time, and the eggshell-walking spouse ultimately gets accused of failing to do enough to organize a smooth life for the hot reactor. Amazingly, for many years, the spouse of a hot reactor lives in a codependent trap, feeling guilty that he or she has indeed somehow "caused" the hot reactor's outbursts.

Their Pitfalls

Eventually, the spouse grows tired of being the target of such outbursts and begins to go numb when dealing with the hot reactor as a defense against the abuse. The spouse justifies withdrawing in this way: "All of this love and support were supposed to help you calm down and act more decently. Given all that I put up with from you, I at least deserve for you to control your temper when dealing with me. This obviously is not working. The deal is off. You have driven me away."

A particularly problematic version of this pattern involves a hot-reacting male physician and his interference-running wife. In such a relationship, the physician often wields tremendous power, evidenced not only by the threat of his outbursts but also by the self-aggrandizement of his work and the "rights" that are his for enduring the stresses of his profession. He may proclaim that, given what he tolerates in his life, he has earned the right to do whatever he likes with his free time, to feel justified in his irritability, and to abdicate any responsibility for contributing to the quality of his home life. Any marriage that revolves around such behavior typically contains power-balancing counterreactions by the "one-down" spouse. Specifically, a wife in such a marriage may express power in her ability to control family relationships and the couple's sexual behavior. The case of Glenn and Sara demonstrates the pain of this process.

Glenn and Sara

Glenn was a plastic surgeon who sought marital therapy because of his frustration with his sexual relationship with his wife of eighteen years, Sara. The comments of each of these spouses sheds a different light on their struggle.

His comments:

"We have not had fun making love in over three years. We do have sex, but it's not much more than masturbation. Sara doesn't kiss me; she doesn't look at me; she doesn't make a sound; she hardly moves her body. She just closes her eyes and waits to get it over with.

"Nothing I have done has worked to make this better. We travel a good bit, but even when we are out of town, supposedly relaxing, she doesn't act relaxed; at least not in our bedroom. I buy her gifts. I've tried giving her massages. I compliment her looks. I take care to keep physically fit and attractive. Nothing works."

Her comments:

"It's true that I do not particularly enjoy making love to Glenn. It's also true that he has tried hard in these past two years to make it better. He has bought me gifts, taken me on trips, and has been more attentive to me than ever before. But I don't feel very sexual when I am with him, and I don't know what to do about it.

"To tell you the truth, I don't know that I want *to do anything about it. Even all of these 'nice' things that Glenn is doing these days are aimed at his getting something that* he *wants, not at anything that I want. This is how it has always been. He works hard to get whatever he wants and doesn't much see—or maybe he just doesn't much care—what other people want.*

"Our life has completely revolved around Glenn's needs and his anger when he doesn't get his way. And he certainly has gotten used to doing it 'his way'—screaming and throwing things if he got frustrated, leaving it to everyone else to clean up the mess caused by his outbursts. Well, that might work in an operating room filled with dutiful nurses, but I've got news for him: It stopped working in this family a long time ago. Problem is, he hasn't even caught on yet as to what has happened in our personal life, and I'm tired of trying to teach him about how to be a good husband and father.

"What's going to happen? I don't know. Maybe a lot. Maybe we'll get a divorce. Maybe nothing at all. I haven't decided. My children are grown-up enough to avoid him. They treat him cordially, and he mistakes that for warmth. Every year one or the other of them asks, 'Why don't you just leave him, Ma?' I guess they love him, but I know that they don't much like him. And neither do I."

Ain't This a Shame

This emotional shutdown threatens the hot reactor with abandonment—a major "violation" of the original relationship contract that promised unending love and acceptance despite the hot reactions. The threatened or actual abandonment at home may occur at the same time the physician is experiencing the disillusionments that come with medical practice. No matter how grandiose a physician's sense of self, he will inevitably be confronted with humbling realities that threaten his sense of omnipotence: death, uncertainty, treatment failures, and his own mistakes—all forcing a revamping of one's sense of power. What happens next for many hot reactors is further self-aggrandizement. In this scenario, grandiosity can be seen as a defense against depression, which can itself be a reaction to the loss of the sense of self.

What do hot reactors do when confronted with their fear of losing both the aggrandized self and the love and acceptance that was "promised" in marriage? They feel ashamed. A gnawing feeling of shame begins to be associated with the relationship. They may feel shame about feeling so needy, shame about being overwhelmed by emotions like sadness, and shame over the fear of being abandoned.

Unfortunately, like one-trick ponies, when hot reactors feel such distress, they reach for their most familiar coping strategy: They get angry. We find that Sam Osherson's comments about angry men fit both male and female hot reactors:

> The closeness of an intimate relationship can awaken a man's early developmental experiences with shame, leaving him feeling dependent, incompetent and awkward in this forbidden territory, and confused over his seemingly conflicting needs. Men can thus be shamed by the depth of soothing they experience in an intimate relationship. . . . many men are so humiliated at their wish to be mothered that they get angry and provoke fights when they feel most in need of help and support.[1]

As feelings of emotional deprivation accumulate in the marriage, such a self-focused hot reactor will typically become more dependent on the applause that comes from work. Grandiosity is bolstered by the admiration and compliance of dependent patients who mirror their most powerful aspects of self, a mirroring that has been shattered in their marriage by the violence of their own hot reactions. We believe that this personal dynamic often underlies the frequently reported finding that, across medical specialties, being needed by their patients is the greatest source of satisfaction for physicians.

Who Is This Helping? Who Is This Hurting?

For these couples, the power struggle stage of the relationship can get very complex and volatile. If the spouse is not a hot reactor, then he or she is likely to settle into depression. Life fills with haunting, difficult-to-answer questions: "Why am I tolerating all of this abuse?" "Maybe I should leave this relationship."

If there are children in the family, the spouse worries about the hot reactor's effect on the kids, especially about actual or feared episodes of physical and verbal abuse at the hands of the hot reactor.

Sometimes spouses of hot reactors are shackled to the relationship not only by their own ambivalence toward their mate, but also by their fear of what the hot reactor might do if they leave. They have seen their mates collapse into periods of desperate depression and clinging and have usually been the targets of the hot reactor's need for bolstering in between long stints of functioning in the Superperson state.

Watch Out!

If the spouse, too, is a hot reactor, the power struggle stage of the relationship can escalate to dangerous degrees. Volatile arguments and physical fighting can punctuate the couple's life together. These couples may alternately batter and cling to each other in an ever-sicker form of dependence and ambivalence about their relationship.

In or Out? I Can't Decide, so I'll Do Nothing

For the hot reactor, an intimate relationship can become an arena filled with frustration and guilt. Frustrations brew in response to the infinite unpredictability and "sloppiness" of day-to-day marriage and family life. Projections and selective perceptions may fuel a misguided notion: "This marriage is the only place that drives me crazy; maybe I should leave." But deeply felt insecurities about love, attachment, and abandonment, coupled with guilt over the episodes of hot reacting, perpetuate the hot reactors' tendency to alternately batter and cling to their mates.

Despite what may seem to be angry indifference, hot reactors do worry about the effect their outbursts are having on their loved ones. Perhaps even more haunting is the fear that these "uncontrollable" episodes will eventually drive their families away.

The reactions and counterreactions can lead such couples into joint emotional shutdown. Remaining open and involved with each other becomes too frustrating and risky. The emotional chaos and desperation that fill these marriages typically lead to the proverbial sentiment "I can't live with you, and I can't live without you." Here, successful renegotiation of the relationship contract is dependent on the hot reactor's learning new, more healthy ways of dealing with anger and the spouse's learning to refuse to fit into a lifestyle that perpetuates this destructive pattern.

Pattern 6: The Island Man or Woman: When Cold Reactors Kill the Love

Here the relationship revolves around an emotionally distanced, obsessive, logical individual who is not comfortable with intimacy and is a fanatic about control. Anyone who is excessively cognitive, rational, perfectionistic, or obsessive-compulsive—and who is bombarded by the stresses of an overwhelming lifestyle—is at risk of developing this coping style. These are people who seem to be islands; they are uncomfortable with physical, verbal, or emotional intimacy. They may actually experience human contact and touch as aversive.

The roots of this pattern might extend to physical traits stemming from childhood. Some researchers have posited that so-called stiff babies—those who are not soothed by cuddling and rocking—actually find physical contact aversive rather than soothing. It has been hypothesized that some babies do not release relaxation-generating endorphins in response to human touch. These stiff babies may accumulate negative relationship experiences that lead them to associate discomfort with human contact. Perhaps the discomfort generalizes to any form of intimacy, and they then learn to focus on their intellect and avoid human contact. As a result, they may never feel comfortable participating intimately with others.

The above hypothesis awaits thorough scientific investigation. However, there is no doubt that people who fit into the *Island* pattern find that responding to and tolerating the needs of others is something they must remind themselves to do. Otherwise, the urge to connect with others may not arise. They simply do not find taking care of others in an intimate way (or being taken care of) comfortable, satisfying, or gratifying.

Their Roles

The contract that serves as the foundation of this relationship typically revolves around the Island's rationality and loneliness. The Island's logical, nonemotional approach to life is at first appealing and stabilizing for his or her mate, who is almost always relatively emotional. The Island's penchants for logic, order, and intellectualization are seen as signs of maturity and, often, intellectual brilliance. These relationships organize around a parent-child dynamic, with the Island in the role of parent.

Psychiatrist Martin Goldberg noted that when the parent-child dynamic occurs in a marriage between a male physician and a nonphysician spouse, the results can be complex.[2] According to Goldberg, when wives in these marriages have a rather hysterical personality type, they may play the pseudochild who gratifies her needs for attention and support by trying to be pretty and charming, or weak and dependent. The physician assumes the role of the father: a strong, protective caretaker for the child-wife. On the surface, his obsessive-compulsive personality type seems to make him immune to emotional storms. This gives him, at least to a hysterical female partner, an aura of strength and protectiveness.

The wife, on the other hand, assumes the role of "caretaker of the emotions" in the relationship. She is the pursuer; the Island is the distancer. The spouse may cling to the notion that this isolated person actually harbors a wealth of unexpressed tenderness and longing. She is touched by the fact that her lonely, brilliant partner sometimes avalanches into depression. Accordingly, the spouse adopts the role of anchor during the storms of depression that inevitably come when the Island is confronted by his or her lack of perfection.

We agree with Goldberg's observation that when it does occur in a medical marriage, this pattern is most likely to involve a male physician in the Island role. We have never counseled a couple in which both individuals were Islands. (If both partners were Islands, all of that isolation probably would prohibit love and romance from ever blossoming into marriage.) However, the Island role is not "male-only" territory. We have treated a number of medical couples in which the female M.D. assumed the Island role in reacting to a more emotional, pursuing husband.

Their Hopes

The fundamental underlying hope of the Island is that his or her mate will always be there, but at a distance. A secondary hope is that the mate will learn to temper his or her emotional style with the organization and rationality that the Island has been role modeling, coaching, teaching, and preaching.

The spouse hopes that, if shown enough nurturing attention, the Island will eventually learn to be comfortable with love and affection. The hope is that the Island will develop into a well-rounded person who can go from brilliant and cognitive to warm and playful.

Their Lifestyle

Life for these couples revolves around critical monitoring by the Island mate or around the Island's seeming indifference to the details of the spouse's life. If the relationship fills with verbalized or implied criticism of the other partner, no aspect of the spouse escapes the Island's scrutiny. The mate's physique, punctuality, organizational abilities, accomplishments, parenting style, extended family relationships, friendships, hobbies, and more are all evaluated and deemed "not quite right— try harder and maybe you'll get it." Ambivalence about whether they themselves are lovable propels Islands into offering conditional love and respect that is never quite earned by other people.

Islands harbor shame over their deeply felt loneliness and vulnerability. By disdaining and ridiculing others, they shift blame for their own pain onto others and momentarily escape their discomfort. In their criticizing, they remain somewhat connected with others; after all, criticism requires that the other person at least be noticed. But this stated or implied criticism also keeps others at a necessary distance.

An Island may eventually stop interacting with loved ones altogether. The silence created by the Island's indifference to everything but his or her own intellectualized pursuits is stifling. These people spend most of their time emotionally or literally isolated from their marriage and family. When not criticizing, they may fail to notice the talents, interests, worries, victories, vulnerabilities, or activities that fill the lives of their loved ones.

Their Pitfalls

Eventually, these become marriages of quiet desperation. The spouse of an Island grows depressed from the lack of intimacy and the conviction that the Island will never change into a comfortable, nurturing partner.

The physician's being in the Island role can lead to a chaotic version of the pursuer-distancer dance. The spouse may attempt to obtain nurturing by assuming a sick and suffering role. But physicians often resent their spouse's problems or concerns. They run out of nurturing in the course of their days of caretaking and come home with an attitude that says "No more problems, please."

In these marriages, this dynamic can get played out to an extreme. According to Goldberg, the more obsessive and detached the physician-husband becomes, the more hysterical the spouse acts.

> He does not prove to be the good father figure his spouse had expected. She is apt to try more and more frantically for his attention and protection by becoming more demanding, developing physical complaints and difficulties, and by increasing emotional disturbance. Her behavior only drives her husband into more obsessive detachment; his detachment feeds her apprehensive weakness and her increasingly frantic demands. The circle is quite complete and quite vicious.[2]

Eventually, many spouses of Islands conclude that their partners are flawed and are *incapable* of expressing warm feelings. They see the Island as suffering the malady experienced by many physicians: "the legacy of life-long emotional constriction so characteristic of compulsive personalities."[3]

Virtually every spouse of an Island whom we have counseled has seriously considered leaving the marriage. These spouses often conclude that their partner is not going to change, due to a lack of either ability or desire. At the same time, they feel shackled to the marriage by their concern for their partner's well-being. Not only are they concerned about their mate's isolation and loneliness, they also fear the Island's capacity for self-destruction.

Despite their seeming indifference to human contact, Islands suffer periods of despair and depression triggered by loneliness and terror when faced with failure or threats of abandonment from their mate. High-powered Islands are especially prone to spend extended periods of time in the Superperson state, only to crash into despondency and depression when faced with a setback or a real or threatened loss. Then, rather than getting angry (the "trick" that is perfected by the hot reactors discussed above), the "Island" bounces back into the Superperson state and goes along his or her preoccupied and distracted way of life.

That the Island might self-destruct if the marriage ends is often a realistic concern. Such people logically question whether or not their life would be worth living if their partner abandoned them. They harbor desperate and primitive feelings of dependency on their loved ones but an equally elemental discomfort when attempting to participate in intimate relationships. These physicians are found to be at greatest risk of suicide.

Such relationships are at risk of settling into an emotional divorce. The couple may remain legally married, but the hope of intimate connection dies. Passion is gone; indifference sets in. They lead separate lives—unless, of course, the Island faces the challenge to learn to show more empathy, compassion, and affection.

References

1. Osherson S. *Wrestling With Love: How Men Struggle With Intimacy, With Women, Children, Parents, and Each Other.* New York, NY: Fawcett Columbine; 1992:179.
2. Goldberg M. Conjoint therapy of male physicians and their wives. *Psychiatr Opin.* 1975;12:19-23.
3. Gabbard GO, Menninger RW. The psychology of postponement in the medical marriage. *JAMA.* 1989;261:2380.

Chapter 13

We've Got a Secret!

Silence maintains control in the face of shame.
—**Sam Osherson, Ph.D., and Steven Kruegerman, Ph.D.**

Pattern 7: Too Mellow to Admit It

We have a whole new generation of medical couples who struggle with a relatively unique dilemma. Similar to the *Ready, Set, Go!* pattern, these couples are typically comprised of two high achievers. But the competition within the marriage is more subtle than obvious and has nothing to do with achievement; it has to do with shame. These partners have an additional clause in their marital dynamic: They have been taught to feel ashamed of such "crass" characteristics as hurrying, competing, workaholism, and being controlling of others. So they try to keep their own such tendencies a secret and subtly compete with each other in efforts to rid themselves of TYABP.

We call this pattern the *Too Mellow to Admit It* medical marriage. Here the marital struggle revolves around each partner's attempt to outdo the other in maintaining at least a semblance of being "laid back 60s style" as they manage the drivenness that comes with their big life.

Their Roles

As in the *Ready, Set, Go!* pattern, these couples are initially attracted to each other's high energy. However, they also share an attraction to the legacies of the late 1960s and early 1970s. Either due to coming of age during this period or through joining with the many members of the emerging generation that idealizes the values and lifestyle of the 1960s, they have embraced the message that people who are "laid back and centered" are healthier than those "poor slobs" who get caught in some materialistic, time-urgent rat race.

These individuals typically possess well-honed social graces and espouse the value of a balanced life. They explicitly and implicitly agree to be partners, using their talents to establish a life that will revolve around the right balance of meaningful work, adequate play, and their abilities to fit into the system without selling out their individuality. With noble intentions, they contract to help each other orchestrate a rich and values-centered life.

Many such couples commit themselves to creating medical practices that are unique in their structure. During a recent speaking engagement in Alaska, we were struck by the seeming "new breed"of physician that predominated: high-powered, superbly educated M.D.s who structured their practices so that they could take every third week off. They and their mates have proudly traded hundreds of thousands of dollars over the span of their careers for free time to enjoy their lives. (Of course, as the spouses of these seemingly mellow physicians pointed out to us, many of those supposedly laid-back docs filled their weeks "off" with such superachiever avocational quests as becoming the perfect fisherman, pilot, snow skier, and so on.)

This is a drastic departure from the mentality that pervaded medicine until recent times. Segraves and Segraves state:

> Forty to fifty years ago, it was not unusual for surgical programs to prohibit married physicians from entering surgical residencies. These educational programs were based on the belief that a residency should occupy the physician's total attention and energy. There was no question but that the future surgeon—once he entered practice—would automatically place the practice of medicine first and marriage second.[1]

And the quality of his personal life last.

While it does appear that work is no longer the primary focus of energy for many contemporary physicians, all is not rosy in these medical marriages. As was discussed in Chapter 2, physicians today expect it all: to be good physicians *and* to enjoy a full and rewarding personal life. Herein lies the seed of conflict in many *Too Mellow to Admit* It marriages.

More so than any other generation of medical marriages or any other medical-marriage pattern, the *Too Mellow to Admit It* couples epitomize the "I deserve to get it all" ethic. Older physicians (late fifties and beyond) came of age when physician-dominated lifestyles were the rule. They counted on (and attained) material success, but they did not put a high priority on actively participating in day-to-day marriage and family life. The young adults currently entering medical school expect less affluence than any previous group of physicians, and the *Too Mellow to Admit* It generation of physicians is now old enough to have tasted of many of the soon-to-be extinct fruits of their labors (such as endlessly escalating incomes).

But these same physicians are young enough to worry about what impact the changes in medicine will have on the remaining chapters of their careers.

These dynamics may lead to clashes between different generations of physicians who try to work together. The aging baby boomer physician, reasoning that he or she has paid his or her dues and thereby earned the right to certain privileges that should come with senior physician status, expects younger M.D.s to take up the baton of excessive devotion to work. But the new generation of physicians, like their Generation X counterparts across professions, is refusing to shape their lives around blind commitment to work. From the outset of their careers, these young physicians are demanding more time for a personal life than have any prior generation of physicians.

Their Hopes

In many ways, these couples have the trickiest dynamics of the eight patterns of medical marriage in our model. Having absorbed the narcissistic lessons of our culture, these high-powered people claim a peculiar version of the right to "have it all." They not only expect success, health, beauty, freedom, fun, and help from each other in overcoming their secret Type A tendencies; they *also* expect their partner to pretend that these Type A tendencies *do not even exist!* For these couples, their drivenness is a dark secret, and they hope and expect that their mate will never see them in that light.

Their Lifestyle

In a nutshell, the *Too Mellow to Admit* It partners try to find a way to live a jam-packed life without showing its effects. They make sure to incorporate diverse interests into their life. They attend the symphony and ballet. They claim to cherish unstructured time. They applaud the successes of colleagues, relatives, and friends. They generally behave in gracious and caring ways, at least in their dealings with the outside world.

What gradually surfaces in the privacy of their relationship is their shared intensity. The other spouse is privy to the secrets they most regret about themselves: perhaps their burning competitiveness, their racial prejudices, their preoccupation with work, their boredom with the day-to-day process of parenting, or their secret wish to leave those glorious cultural and artistic functions at intermission out of a desire to move on to something more stimulating or urgent (like paperwork!).

Their Pitfalls

As their marriage progresses and the stresses of their lifestyle escalate, the partners in a *Too Mellow to Admit It* medical marriage begin accusing each other of being responsible for the lifestyle that is driving them: "*You* were the one who wanted this big house. Now *I* have to worry about paying for it. Of course I'm angry!"

Counteraccusations accumulate: "If we had left it to *me*, we would still be living on one income and banking the other. I remind you that *I* was still a semihippie when we met. *You* were the one who decided: 'We have the money, let's send the kids to private school.' Now we're working ourselves to death to support *your* notion of keeping up with your fraternity brothers."

In small ways, these couples often resort to shaming each other whenever any TYABP is shown. An outburst of profanity by one of them at a slow-moving driver is met with a look of disgust and a sigh of resignation. Irritability about lack of punctuality is met with passive-aggressive moseying: "Just stopping to smell the roses. For god's sake, don't be in such a hurry!"

Sometimes silent competition over who can be the more nurturing parent revolves around this shaming game. A dual-physician couple we treated noticed that when either of them got irritable, the other acted more patient and nurturing with the children. While this made for a soothing moment in the family dynamic, it felt like a passive-aggressive attack on the irritated partner. In many ways the nurturing partner was parenting "at" the irritated one: "Look how laid back I am. Why don't you just chill out, get out of your hurry flurry, and come back to earth?" Such behavior was simultaneously nurturing to the children and critical of the partner.

These couples let each other know that TYABP is unacceptable. What they fail to realize is that their disgust with TYABP is more a rebellion against their own internal struggles than a reaction to any outrageous behavior of their partner. This becomes a process of projection. Each partner's internal struggle gets projected onto their perceptions of the other, and the couple then enacts the conflicts that one (and usually both) of them feel.

The pitfall for these couples comes during the midlife push to come to terms with one's integrated self. These people grow tired and resentful of trying to be someone they're not. This does not mean that they want permission to become wildly out-of-control superachievers. By definition, these are people whose sensibilities prevent them from settling into denial. The partners in a *Too Mellow to Admit It* medical marriage simply grow tired of having another person relentlessly monitor them and criticize their values. As one of our physician-patients stated:

I looked in the mirror this morning and finally saw who I am. I'm a forty-nine-year-old physician who is a quasi-Type A. I'm a former flower child, and it's time for me to accept the fact that the operative word in this sentence is 'former.' The truth is that I'm a Republican, rather mate-rialistic, impatient with people who are incompetent, and a person who would rather watch a basketball game than attend the ballet.

But I also realized that I'm a good and loving father, a damned good doctor, and a man who is willing to work hard to help our society save our planet. I am not a laid-back earth mother. I am not a self-absorbed monster. I'm who I am.

My wife fancies herself to be so different than I am in all of these ways. Because she's an artist, she figures that she's Miss Mellow. What a joke! Try interrupting her when she's in the midst of a 'creative flurry,' as she calls it. She'll bite your head off. But then again, that's just 'an artist's temperament.' If I'm grouchy after staying up all night on call, then I'm being 'a typical Type A physician.' No 'artistic license' here!

Which gets me to another point: I'm sick and tired of her taking some unrealistic moral high ground with me. I am freaked out over what might happen in medicine during the upcoming years. I'm afraid that the government and the insurance industry are going to ruin my profession and my career. My wife seems to take pride in advertising what a Democrat she is. She proselytizes, saying, 'We can certainly live on less,' and, 'Something's got to be done about the system as it is,' and, 'Let's not forget our obligation to others.' She acts like we're back in college, marching on Washington to protest the Vietnam War.

What she seems to have forgotten is that I am not Richard Nixon, for God's sake! When all of these noble sentiments of hers start hitting home, we'll see how 'actualized' she feels. We can't even talk about this without arguing. She claims I'm just taking a position. I am taking a position: I'm scared!

This is complicated stuff. I agree that some things have to change in medicine. And I am willing to be a part of the change. But my worries are more basic than she seems to understand. Will we be able to educate our kids the way we plan to? Will we be able to afford her working as an artist? She barely makes any money. How about our house? Or helping our parents during their retirement? Or funding our own retirement?

I feel like I am being more grown-up and realistic than I ever have been in my lifetime, and I can't talk with my wife about what I see without getting labeled in some pejorative way. I'm sick and tired of being told to be someone I'm not. I'm almost fifty years old; it's time to stop struggling with my wife about who I am.

Final Words

Each of the patterns of medical marriage we have discussed thus far begins as a soothing island of refuge that holds the hope of providing both partners with a potent source of nurturing and fulfillment. Growth in each of these relationship patterns is complicated not only by the stress of medical careers but also by one form or another of high-powered coping and one version or another of an unrealistic relationship contract born of narcissistic expectations.

What can be done to prevent the seemingly inevitable consequences?

Reference
1. Segraves K, Segraves RT. When the physician's marriage is in trouble. *Med Aspects Hum Sexuality*. June 1987:148-149.

Chapter 14

Managing Anger & Conflict

This has been far more difficult than I thought it would be. My husband is so angry so much of the time. If we talk, all he talks about is how frustrated he is with what's going on at the hospital and in his practice. And if I complain, I become the target of his rage.

—**Myra,** wife of physician, Jim

What am I supposed to do? I'm fed up with incompetence, I'm bombarded with frustration, I'm tired of people trying to tell me what to do. Yes, I am angry, and yes, I do let it fly! What other choice do I have? If I don't express it, I'll explode. Well, I already do explode; but if I hold it in, I'll explode worse.

—**Jim,** physician

Throughout this book, we have emphasized one key to staying stress-resilient: You must proactively work to maintain positive, loving connection with each other. Targeted strategies for doing just that will follow shortly.

Here, we want to address a second key to stress resilience: Both at work and home, you must learn to manage anger and conflict without damaging your relationships.

Two indisputable facts are important here. First, no ongoing relationship escapes periods of conflict. If you authentically relate to another person across time, you will regularly discover differences in what each of you thinks, feels, needs, or wants. How you manage these times of conflict will either bolster your trust in and respect for each other, or damage your relationship.

Second, damaged relationships in any important life arena tend to lead to negative emotional consequences (like anger) that can generalize to other life arenas. Put simply, negative emotions tend to be "contagious." We repeatedly find evidence for this phenomenon. For example, the quality of a physician's home life does, indeed, have a great impact on his or her stress resilience at work. And the quality of work relationships clearly affects one's home life. For these reasons, learning to manage anger and conflict is an aspect of beating stress together that has benefits in both arenas. (If our experiences are any indication, this is a timely issue. Recently, the journal *The Physician Executive* invited us to write a two-part series titled "The Angry Physician."[1,2] Nothing has ever brought us more consulting business.)

So What's New?

Physicians have always lived pressure-packed lives, and prolonged stress can lead to short fuses and strained tolerance. That's nothing new. But, historically, physicians also enjoyed high levels of control. As rulers of their workplaces, they enjoyed high levels of autonomy. In other words, they lived in high-demand/high-control stress paradigms—the kind of stress that is quite energizing and motivating.

How times have changed! As the practice of medicine has been reshaped by the intrusion of business agendas, two things have happened: Demands have increased, and control has been stripped from physicians. Now, more than ever before, practicing medicine means encountering high-demand/low-control stressors, the type that researcher Robert Karasek identified as being most irritating and most toxic to physical and emotional well-being.[3] In our opinion, the question is not whether you will face the challenge to appropriately manage anger and conflict; *the question is, how is what you're doing working!*

The Rising Costs of Anger

Health psychologist Timothy Smith of the University of Utah reminds us that what we typically refer to simply as "anger" actually involves three distinct phenomena:

- Anger—an unpleasant emotional experience that may range from irritation to rage.
- Hostility—the tendency to wish harm on others or to feel anger toward others. Simply put, hostility is a set of negative attitudes or beliefs that others will probably mistreat, frustrate, or provoke you, and therefore are not to be trusted.
- Aggression—overt behavior that typically involves attacking, destructive, or hurtful actions.[4]

The three flavors of anger interrelate: If you get stuck in the habit of being angry, the odds increase that you will develop hostile, cynical attitudes that will lead you to act unnecessarily aggressively. Three things are then likely to happen.

First, if you mismanage anger, you will lose your ability to differentiate one emotion from another. Some high-powered people are like one-trick ponies: They show anger whenever they feel anything. If they feel challenged, they act angry. If they feel scared, they act angry. If they feel insecure, they act angry. If they feel sad, they act angry.

Next, mismanaging anger diminishes your ability to deal with others effectively. As we mentioned earlier, high-powered people often live in a surprising paradox: despite their intimidating style, they secretly feel helpless and vulnerable in relationships. Typically, their aggressiveness and defensiveness have to do with deeply felt anxieties and insecurities about their own worth and about their ability to deal with others. But their behavior complicates, rather than soothes, their tensions.[5] Their relationship style creates circumstances that leave them feeling victimized because they give others the power to stir their own extreme reactions, which leave them feeling ineffectual.

Mismanaged hostility is also one of the most dangerous risks to your health. Hostility researchers Redford and Virginia Williams warn that, for the chronically hostile person, "getting angry is like taking a small dose of poison—arsenic, for example—every day of your life."[6] In fact, those who score high on measures of chronic hostility tend to die young from all causes of mortality. Highly hostile people are more accident prone, engage in more acts of aggression or violence, and tend to develop unhealthy lifestyles. The high-hostile are also at elevated risk of developing certain illnesses, including heart disease, high blood pressure, ulcerative colitis, and others.

Should I Show My Anger?

We do not intend to imply that healthy people never show anger, or that, to be a happy medical couple, you must learn to live in perpetual harmony. On the contrary, the eminent marital researcher John Gottman documented that a major feature of long-lasting marriages is recurrent periods of conflict.[7] But healthy couples learn to argue constructively. Gottman's research underscores the importance of learning to express anger in distinctive ways:

- Stay focused on the issue, not on name-calling
- Defuse anger with signs of affection (a loving look, touch, or warm gesture)
- Use humor in a positive way (laugh with each other, not at each other)

If you justify anger outbursts with the notion that it's better to express anger than it is to hold it inside, you're making a serious mistake. The truth is that an unbridled expression of anger does only one thing—it makes you more angry. The more frequently you act angry, the more likely it is that you will feel angry.

What Can I Do About This?

Start by examining the function that anger plays in your life. Anger serves high-powered people in many ways. Anger can fuel motivation. It can be a defense against such painful feelings as fear or sadness. It can also signal that some forceful action is needed to deal with a stressful situation. As in other aspects of controlling yourself, even during the uncontrollable times of your life, the goal is to control what happens once you *get* angry.

Next, take stock of whether you have a problem. In addition to listening to feedback from others regarding your anger management style, it's helpful to evaluate your relationships using the following scale. This scale is based on the concept that, in any ongoing relationship, disagreements are inevitable; the task is to prevent disagreements from solidifying into conflict.

The *Stages of Conflict* scale that follows can help you to do two things. First, this is a quick way to assess the status of any relationship on the continuum of healthy disagreement to toxic conflict. Second, the scale outlines specifically how disagreements can escalate into conflict. Remember that, due to differences of opinion, needs, or interpretations of facts, disagreements are inevitable in any ongoing relationship. If you can simply agree to disagree and avoid locking into defensive competition with each other, you can deal with whatever problem faces you without damaging your relationship.

But, as can be seen in the scale below, trouble starts when you start to see the other person as b*eing the problem*. This change in perspective leads to defensiveness, withholding of positive regard, and competitiveness. Soon, a win-lose mentality sets in, and the relationship becomes toxic.

Stages of Conflict Scale[8]

Check items that apply to your organization or family. Total the checks at each stage of conflict.

Stage 1: Agreeing to Disagree

- ☐ Willing to meet and discuss facts
- ☐ A cooperative spirit prevails
- ☐ Issues can be discussed without involving personalities
- ☐ The language used is specific
- ☐ There is a sense of optimism

☐ There is a "live and let live" attitude
☐ Parties are able to stay in the present tense
☐ Solutions dominate your management efforts
Total Stage 1 Characteristics: _____

Stage 2: Conflict Begins to Heat Up the System
☐ A competitive attitude predominates
☐ Talk about problems targets people as being the problem
☐ Discussion frequently involves use of statements like "They," "You always," and "He never"
☐ A "cover your rear" attitude predominates
☐ Generalized language is used
☐ There is an emphasis on winners and losers
☐ There is a cautious atmosphere when issues are discussed
☐ Individuals are making efforts to look good
Total Stage 2 Characteristics: _____

Stage 3: Dysfunctional Patterns Solidify
☐ Attempts are made to eliminate others from problem-solving process
☐ Obvious leaders or spokespersons have emerged for different sides
☐ There is a sense of "holy mission" on the part of certain individuals
☐ There has been a loss of middle ground
☐ There is an intention to hurt
☐ A choosing of sides has occurred
☐ The collective good has become identified with a set of special interests
☐ There is a sense that the conflict will never end with only one-sided, all-or-nothing options being proposed
Total Stage 3 Characteristics _____

Adapted from: Waitley D. *How to Handle Conflict and Manage Anger: Action Guide.* Niles, Ill: Nightingale-Conant Corp; 1995. With modifications by Wayne and Mary Sotile, 1998.

If your responses to the *Stages of Conflict* scale indicate that your relationship is drifting toward Stage 2, take stock and commit yourself to not engaging in the sorts of behaviors that will push you into Stage 3 conflict. Tips on how to do this will close this chapter. On the other hand, if you are already locked into a Stage 3 conflict, consider consulting a counselor trained in conflict management to help you to resolve your issues without further damaging your relationship.

What Is Your Anger About?

Some people are lucky. They are able to abruptly switch from being generally angry to being generally calm. Shocked by a life-changing experience, a religious conversion, or a brush with death, for example, they undergo a global change and become more loving and accepting of others.

We say that these folks are lucky because they experience an unusual form of psychological change: their emotional change makes it relatively easy for them to subsequently change their attitudes and behaviors. Simply put, because they no longer feel anger as frequently as they used to, it's relatively easy for them to not act aggressively or think hostile thoughts.

Of course, this is not the way it goes for most of us. As one of our patients put it:

Telling me to feel peaceful and compassionate as a way of controlling my temper, that's stupid. If I felt peaceful and compassionate, I wouldn't need to control my temper! The problem is that I do not feel peaceful or compassionate. Most of the time, I feel rushed and aggravated. So, what am I supposed to do?

Most of us have to approach anger management in a systematic, situation-by-situation manner that is typical of how psychological and behavioral changes tend to occur. Recall the change process we outlined earlier: Attitudinal change leads to behavioral change, and behavioral practice eventually leads to emotional change. If you are willing to bear through the awkwardness of changing, you can behave yourself into developing the habit of adaptively handling anger and effectively negotiating conflict.

Break Up the Dominoes. Learning to manage conflict without damaging your relationships rests on your ability, as an individual, to control your anger. Think of anger reactions as being the last dominoes in a stress progression.[9] If you can change even a few of the "dominoes"—the specific ways you fuel angry reactions—negotiating your conflicts will be infinitely easier to do. Start by noticing what fuels your feelings.

Our counseling experiences with thousands of people suggest that, if you are chronically angry, it is likely that you are suffering from some combination of three syndromes:

- Your anger signals an ongoing struggle with some disappointment or loss from the past.
- Anger flares because you are dissatisfied with some major aspect of your present life.
- Anger is the by-product of your personality-based coping patterns.

Disappointments and Losses. Experiencing loss is an unavoidable part of living, and loss stirs grief reactions. Simplistically put, healthy grieving moves through the stages of shock, denial, anger, despair, and resolution.

When you pause to think about it, you may be saddened to realize just how much you have lost during your life. Included here are the obvious losses: deaths of loved ones or friends, lost friendships, health problems, or failures. These dramatic losses are typically identified and openly grieved, and acknowledging them usually leads to support, relief, and healing.

But most of us also suffer various "disenfranchised" losses. These typically go unrecognized and unexpressed, and, therefore, tend not to heal. Included here are more subtle losses: loss of your youth; loss of valued opportunities like spending more time with your family when you and they were younger; loss of dreams that did not come true; loss of the ways it used to be during simpler times; or loss of fun and passion in some areas of your life—like your work.

If your grief remains unexpressed or unsoothed, you can become "stuck" in one of its stages. Furthermore, grieving major losses typically unfolds over years, not months. Anyone who loses a cherished loved one knows how true this is. Just because some loss occurred in the distant past, don't assume that adjusting is necessarily finished.

Health care professionals are especially prone to accumulate unresolved grief over the deaths of patients. Unfortunately, the world does not recognize physician grief. When was the last time anyone expressed sympathy or offered you special, nurturing care when one of your patients died? To the contrary, we repeatedly hear from physicians how traumatizing it is when they are openly blamed and shamed by superiors or aggrieved loved ones after the death of a patient.

The question here is: What losses have you experienced that have been particularly difficult to endure, and how are you currently coping with these? If your anger signals unfinished grieving, then you must allow yourself to complete the process. This means finding a safe relationship in which you can talk about what you are feeling. Expressing painful emotions and getting support not only lessens grief, it also prevents the physical complications to health that can come from suppressing negative emotions.

Let yourself feel and talk about your losses. You might find it helpful to write out your feelings, expressing what you appreciated and regretted about the relationship, person, or situation that you lost. Remember: grief is an emotional process that dissipates if it is fully experienced. Don't be afraid of your painful emotions. Geared with the support of others and with a nurturing and self-accepting attitude, let yourself grieve until you are relieved.

Maybe I'm Just Not Satisfied. Anger does not always have to do with grief over what is past. Some people are angry about their here-and-now struggles that come from dissatisfaction with the situations, relationships, or processes that create their life territory.

One obvious way to lessen your anger is to create a life territory that is more to your liking. You might need to find the courage to change where you live, how you live, or whom you deal with. This requires that you accept that eliminating toxic situations, processes, or people from your life is not necessarily the same as running from your problems. More often, it's about defending your right to live a more healthy, meaningful life.

Of course, this is not always possible. Some stresses can't be eliminated. You may suffer from something (such as an illness) or from some relationship (such as with one of your loved ones) that is not changeable. In these circumstances, rather than changing the external causes of your anger, you must learn to change your internal reactions. This involves taking an honest look at how your personality drives you into anger.

Personality Scripting. Certain situations are especially likely to stir anger for people driven by each of the personality scripts referred to earlier. Review the following table and note what applies to you.

Personality Drivers and Anger

If your personality compels you to:	You will likely experience anger in the following situations:
Be Strong	When you are challenged; during interpersonal conflict; when you are asked to talk about your inner thoughts or feelings
Be Perfect	When your quests for perfection are encumbered by your own or another's lack of perfection; when you perceive someone as challenging your control
Please Others	When you are accused of behaving selfishly
Try Hard	When you are accused of being lazy or of not having tried hard enough; when you deal with others who do not seem to share your value for hard work
Hurry Up	When you are forced to slow your urgent pace because of some unexpected factor—such as someone else moving slowly, or due to your own limitations
Be Careful	When you are asked to trust that another will be competent or nurturing

Once you identify the sorts of situations that are most likely to stir your anger, beware. Accept that some of these situations are probably inevitable parts of your life, and remind yourself to take extra care to remain mindful of your thoughts and behaviors during these circumstances.

Calming the Storm Within

One foundation of anger management is controlling what you say to yourself about other people. Psychologist Robert Alan emphasizes that anger often signals a threat to an underlying need and occurs as a result of what he calls an anger-judgment complex, whereby anger is fueled either by the judgment that you are being done an injustice or the judgment that your stress is happening due to someone's incompetence.[10]

A judgment of injustice might involve seeing the situation that you face as being unfair, improper, wrong, or the result of someone being inconsiderate or biased in dealing with you.

A judgment of incompetence might involve seeing your stress as being caused by another's shortcomings, such as stupidity, laziness, inadequacy, or lack of qualifications.

This way of understanding your anger leads to three key guidelines for disrupting anger reactions.

When you first notice yourself becoming angry you should:

- Identify your underlying needs at that moment.
- Recognize and counter your own judgments.
- Provide yourself with nonangry alternative ways of coping with the stress at hand and of satisfying your underlying needs.

We close this chapter with discussion of two general strategies for controlling your personal anger reactions and eight specific strategies for managing interpersonal conflict.

Anger Management Strategy 1: Use Empathy to Counter Judgments

Counter your judgments by forcing yourself to charitably put yourself in the other person's place. Develop the habit of reminding yourself that others are doing the best they can to cope with their world, given who they are and what they have learned from their own experiences.

For example, let's say that you are stuck in a slowly moving checkout line in a grocery store. You notice that the cashier seems to be taking her time in checking out each customer. She moves slowly, chats with each customer, and generally seems to be in no particular hurry to move the line along.

Your reflexive reaction to this situation might be anger-fueling thoughts such as:

"This jerk could care less how long she takes to check us out! Just because she has this dead-end job, she probably thinks that the rest of us have nothing better to do than to stand here and take her foolishness. I swear, I'm sick and tired of taking this kind of foolishness from people!"

Notice that these thoughts are filled with judgments. They suggest that the checkout clerk is purposely persecuting the customers with her incompetence and with her lackadaisical attitude.

A more empathic and self-controlled way of reacting to the same situation might be:

"This line is not moving! That checkout clerk is a slow worker. This aggravates me.

"Okay. Now, let's see. I am angry, but I guess I do have a choice about how I think and act right now. I could decide that this young woman is doing the best that she can. Maybe she's just a hard-working kid who is not very bright at math. Maybe she's just trying to learn how to be a good worker. We all had to start someplace. I can appreciate that; I remember how I fumbled through my first job.

"I might as well find a way to enjoy myself as much as I can while I wait. Maybe I'll use this time to practice relaxing. Maybe I'll just read one of these junk tabloids that I don't usually buy. Maybe I'll have a nice daydream. . . ."

Use the following list of self-statements to help control your internal responses during frustrating situations. See such situations as opportunities to practice anger control. Remind yourself that developing the habit of reacting to others with empathy rather than criticism will serve you well.

Managing Anger: Coping Statements[11]

- "No point in blaming. I'll try a new strategy."
- "I may not like it, but he/she is probably doing his/her best right now."
- "I have a choice about how I react right now."
- "Is this worth dying for?"
- "Will this matter five years from now?"
- "If I am still angry about this tomorrow, I'll deal with it then."
- "I am free to want what I want, but he or she is free to be different from me."
- "I am not in charge of the world."
- "Anger will not get me what I want."
- "Acting angry is not the same as showing that I care."
- "Calmness is not the same as weakness."
- "There is power in calmness."
- "It's time to relax."
- "Let me ask, rather than tell."
- "I'll listen, rather than talk."
- "This is interesting; let me try to figure it out."
- "I can feel strongly and act calmly."
- "Remember to laugh."
- "I'm in charge of how I react, not him/her."
- "How big is this issue, compared to the size of my life?"
- "Being in a hurry just makes me irritable and not nice to be around."
- "I deserve to enjoy."
- "Hostility is bad for my health."

- "My need to control others is fueled by my own insecurities."
- "It takes real strength and maturity to show love and kindness."
- "This is just a drop of water in a waterfall."

Anger Management Strategy 2: Control Your Behaviors

The next step in managing anger is not psychological; it's behavioral. Even if you seem unable to control your thinking and if your anger is flowing, you will preserve your health and your relationships if you block your urge to act aggressively. This is not only tactful, it's also wise. The aforementioned health risks of chronic hostility are attenuated if aggression is tempered. That means that even if you cannot manage your angry emotions or your hostile thoughts, you can keep from doing harm to yourself and to others if you learn to behave in ways that are not aggressive. For example, researchers have found that modifying your style of speech when having a conflict lessens strain on your heart, even if you are highly angry or frustrated during the conflict.[12,13]

We have worked with countless high-powered people who have benefited markedly from simply learning to differentiate assertion from aggression. In doing so, they have reclaimed their personal power and control in their dealings with difficult people and difficult situations. Doing so requires that you pay particular attention to six aspects of your communication style:

1. your verbal behaviors
2. your nonverbal sounds
3. your voice quality, tone, and volume
4. your hand and arm gestures
5. your facial expressions
6. your body movements

What follows is a list anger-fueling mistakes to be avoided in each of these six categories.

Ways to Fuel Anger[14]

General Category	Specific Examples
Verbal Behaviors	Cursing
	Giving unwanted advice
	Criticizing
	Threatening
	Blaming
	Exaggerating
	Giving ultimatums
	Being sarcastic
	Refusing to discuss the topic

Nonverbal Sounds	Sighing
	Moaning
	Grunting
	Groaning
Voice Quality, Tone, and Volume	Shouting
	Tense, overly controlled
	Mumbling
	Snickering
	Whining
	Flatness, suggesting disinterest
Hand and Arm Gestures	Balling fist
	Pointing a finger
	Shaking a fist
	Folding arms
	Placing hands on hips
	Waving hand, suggesting dismissal
	Pounding or tapping table
	Chopping motion
Facial Expressions	Rolling eyes
	Refusal to make eye contact
	Narrowing eyes
	Grimacing in disgust or disbelief
	Raising eyebrows
	Frowning
	Scowling
Body Movements	Shaking head, indicating "No, no!"
	Shrugging shoulders
	Foot tapping
	Turning away
	Pacing
	Kicking
	Pushing or grabbing

Unfortunately, once we are angry, most of us lose sight of our actions and the impact we are having on others. Often, we express anger in ways that simply perpetuate angry reactions from others, and our own anger reactions escalate. Listening to an audiotape or watching a video of yourself as you deal with a frustrating situation can be an invaluable, sobering experience. This is what happened to Charles when he watched a video replay of a family therapy session in which he angrily criticized his wife and son. "*I* got scared looking at *myself* on that tape," he said sadly. "No wonder my family avoids me whenever things get tense!"

Use the following scale to rate yourself and your partner(s) on anger-generating versus anger-minimizing behaviors.

Angry Behaviors Scale*

Rate yourself on each behavior by placing an "X" where you generally fall on the continuum.

Anger Generators	During a conflict, I most often:	Anger Minimizers
Use disrespectful tones or behaviors	_____	Show respect
Don't look at the other person	_____	Make eye contact
Make unreasonable demands	_____	Focus on practical solutions
Act like I need to be right	_____	Keep an open mind
Pass judgments	_____	Suspend judgments
Use sarcasm, humiliation, attacks, threats	_____	Use an even, calm, but firm tone
Touch or get too close	_____	Maintain appropriate distance
Use aggressive gestures	_____	Use neutral, open gestures
Send mixed messages	_____	Send consistent messages
Show favoritism	_____	Act fairly
Show impatience or act bored	_____	Use active listening skills
Act inflexibly	_____	Act flexibly
Interrupt	_____	Allow reasonable venting
Use negative words	_____	Use positive phrases
Reject the person	_____	Focus on behaviors
Constantly override decisions	_____	Encourage collaboration
Fail to follow through	_____	Follow through on promises
Lie	_____	Be honest
Don't respond to individual needs	_____	Treat others as individuals

*Modified from: Staver M. *21 Ways to Diffuse Anger and Calm People Down.* Boulder, Colo: CareerTrack Pub; 1997.

A number of strategies for better controlling anger can be gleaned from the above information. First, share the information in the *Ways to Fuel Anger* list and the *Angry Behaviors* scale with your mate. Ask for feedback about your style of communicating during disagreements. Try not to get defensive when hearing this feedback. It is not our purpose here to start another argument! We simply want to help you to develop a realistic picture of yourself. You can then use this picture as a guideline for changing.

Next comes the hard part: *You must practice behaving differently.* Once again, review the tables in this chapter, and, this time, take note of alternatives to ineffectual behaviors in each of the major categories. Then *practice* these more controlled ways of acting. Periodically tape-record your conversations at home and work (with everyone' permission, of course), and then review the tape to listen for changes in your style.

Finally, we recommend that you explicitly state your commitment to learn to negotiate your differences without damaging your relationship. Our work with couples who have suffered from mismanaged anger or conflict has led us to believe that it's never too late to benefit from positive change. If you sincerely apologize to your partner for past, inappropriate behavior, commit yourself to changing, and, indeed, follow through, you can generate new levels of trust, self-respect, and family health.

Managing Conflict Without Damaging Your Relationships

Managing personal anger reactions is necessary but not sufficient if you want to build a stronger relationship. You must also learn to effectively deal with each other during the most difficult times of conflict. Eight specific guidelines can help you to resolve differences without hurting your relationships, both at home and at work.

1. Practice Being an Effective Emotional Manager. You will more effectively deal with even the most aggravating situation or person if you are in reasonable control of your overall emotional and stress levels. On the other hand, even a minor irritant can trigger a full-blown anger reaction when you are already overly stressed.

Practicing overall stress management naturally leads to better anger management. If you know your personality-based coping patterns, you will recognize high-risk situations and clarify your underlying needs in those situations. If you control your thinking, you will not turn frustrations into full-blown bouts of anger. Finally, learning to slow down and relax is a key way to calm the psychological and physical swirls that occur during an anger reaction.

2. Respect Your Physiology. When it comes to managing anger, some people are at a disadvantage. Recall our earlier discussion about hot reactors: If you tend to have exaggerated fight-or-flight reactions and impoverished calming reactions, it is especially important to pay attention to choices that affect your baseline stress levels. Beware of stimulants like caffeine, nicotine, and simple sugars. These can magnify the reactions of an already-existing supercharged nervous system. Also remember that doing and thinking more than one thing at once activates the stress response. Regularly take breaks to clear your mind and wash stress out of your body with exercise or relaxation.

3. Learn to Detach. You can detach yourself from a situation or person that is making you angry by learning to relax and depersonalize. In your mind's eye, pretend that you are watching a movie of you and the person with whom you are interacting. Pretend that you are in the audience, calmly watching the two of you up on the screen. This allows you to experience the interaction from a position that is one step removed, a place where it is much easier to control your emotions.

4. Listen to Yourself. At the same time that you are depersonalizing the situation with imagery, control your self-talk. Use anger managing coping statements like those listed above.

5. Strike While the Iron is Warm. We reiterate what we mentioned earlier: Whenever possible, it is wise to wait until your anger calms before responding to another. Truly powerful and assertive people choose their times for dealing with conflict. Use your own good judgment about when you will be at your best to negotiate a complex issue. Remember *not* to strike while the iron is hot. A good formula to follow in this regard is to:
   a. Call time out before responding.
   b. Schedule a time with the person to follow up.
   c. Collect your thoughts and your emotions.
   d. Rehearse how you will deal with the conflict.
   e. Meet with the other person.

6. Deal With One Issue at a Time. Resist the temptation to let anger about one issue lead you into showering the other person with related issues. Remember that any issue important enough to make you angry deserves its own discussion. If a new issue surfaces during your conflict, flag it and apply strategy 5.

7. Start Early. Here, as in many aspects of medicine, the best choice is prevention. Don't wait until you or another person has an outburst before talking about what is happening in your relationship. Use the information in the *Ways to Fuel Anger* table (page 233) to notice subtle signs of anger or irritation in your own or others' behavior. Likewise, if you suspect that someone is upset, ask about it. Offer to help, to simply listen, or to discuss the issue at hand. If you notice yourself showing signs of upset, talk with the person involved. Don't wait. In this way, you can help disrupt domino progressions that otherwise lead to angry outbursts.

8. Negotiate Your Differences Without Damaging Your Relationships. Conflict has been defined as a situation in which two or more people cannot agree on the actions that one person takes, or that one person doesn't want the other to take. When you think of it this way, conflict clearly signals the need to negotiate, not to avoid.

In their helpful book *Getting to Yes,* authors Roger Fisher and William Ury outline a number of practical guidelines for successfully negotiating resolution of conflict in any relationship.[15] Knowing these guidelines can help you manage yourself during difficult discussions.

First, when you experience conflict, remember to separate the person from the problem. Work to create an "us versus the problem" attitude and avoid locking into a "me versus you" mentality. You can do this by using several simple communication strategies:

a. Stroke the Person and Show a Leap of Faith That You Will Resolve the Problem at Hand. *Example:* "I know you're doing what you think is best. I never question your integrity or the fact that you will do whatever you believe will be helpful. I trust that we will be able to resolve this, even though we disagree about what would be the most helpful thing to do. This really is bothering me, though, and I appreciate your willingness to work through this with me."

b. Validate the Other Person's Perceptions. *Example:* "When I put myself in your shoes, I can understand why you must think or feel what you do. Your points are well made and well received. I see things somewhat differently, but I can understand your perspective, too."

c. Focus on the Problem at Hand. Don't Blame or Create a Catastrophe. *Example:* "This is a serious problem. But I know we will find a way to resolve it."

d. Emphasize Where You Agree. *Example*: "We really do think about this in some ways that differ. But we agree more than we disagree. We seem to agree that (a) this is a problem that we need to cooperate in solving; (b) we care enough about our relationship to want to resolve this; and (c) we share the opinion[s] that [fill in the blank] might be helpful."

e. Apologize.   This is not the same as admitting fault or minimizing the point that you are trying to get across. This is simply saying that you are sorry you are having this conflict: a very powerful way to calm otherwise disturbed waters in any relationship.

Example: "I'm sorry that we're going through this right now. I know that neither of us likes it when we argue." Or: "I'm really sorry that we're having this problem with [fill in the blank]. It's not very pleasant for either of us to have to deal with this."

f. Listen.   In resolving conflict, it is important to spend at least as much time listening as you do talking or thinking about what you are planning to say. Try to learn why that person's position on the issue at hand is so important to him or her. Listen for feelings or fears that might underlie the other person's stance. Let the other person know that you have heard what he or she has expressed. By doing so, you will lower the other's defensiveness. Remember: When we are not heard, we tend to repeat what we just said, only this time louder and more forcefully. We also get defensive in proportion to how misunderstood we feel. On the other hand, once we're convinced that we've been heard and understood, we calm down and become open to learning.

Example: "Okay. Let me tell you what I'm hearing as I listen to you. It seems as if you've been feeling that I have not been taking care of my fair share of our household responsibilities. It sounds as if my behavior has been giving you the message 'I don't care what you feel; my stress is more important than your stress' and that you have understandably felt hurt by that message. I also hear that you care enough to talk with me about this.

"Am I following you so far? Am I missing any important pieces of what you are thinking or feeling?"

As you give feedback, be sure to assume an "I" position rather than a blaming position. Even if you are sharing a negative observation, frame your feedback positively. Also, make suggestions regarding how you might be willing to cooperate in changing your part of the process that contributes to the problem that you are identifying.

Example 1: "I think it's true that I sometimes shut down when I feel tension between us; I shut you out. I know that I often seem to pout and that I have not been interested in sex lately. I also know that this bothers you. I think that what we're going through is hard on both of us. I'm sorry that we're having these problems. When you raise your voice and use angry words during our arguments, it really bothers me, and the way I react seems to hurt you.

"I'm willing to try not to shut out communication when I'm hurt or angry. I'd also be willing to go to counseling with you to get some pointers on how we might communicate better. It would mean a lot to me if we could learn a different way of dealing with each other at times like this. I'm willing to do my part, and I know that it will help me do my part if you will learn not to shout when we have a disagreement."

Example 2: "I know that the way I act sometimes irritates you. Things have been tense around here, and I know that I'm pretty stressed. I want to understand your side of this, if you'd like to talk about it. We're partners in this, and I want have a good working relationship with you."

These communication strategies help you to focus on underlying interests, not on positions. Conflicts usually have to do with both parties "posturing": They rigidly assume some position and then do battle from that position even if it does not fully and accurately represent the issues beneath the surface of their attempts to negotiate with each other.

We will use an anecdote from our own relationship (when our two daughters were younger) as an example of this factor.

Wayne: *Let's get a baby-sitter and go out to eat at that new Italian restaurant.*

Mary *(hesitating): I'm not sure I feel like doing that.*

Wayne *(impatient and defensive): Why not? I know that the baby-sitter is available; she told me that she isn't working evenings at her other job this week.*

Mary: *I know she's available. I just don't know . . . I don't exactly feel like doing it.*

Wayne: *Look, I'm Italian, and Italians like to eat Italian food. It seems like you never cook Italian food anymore, and I feel like eating Italian food. I don't understand why you are being so hardheaded about this.*

Mary: *For God's sake! We now have an international crisis on our hands! All right. Let's go eat Italian food. I don't want you to die from spaghetti deprivation. Maybe you should have married a nice little Italian girl who cooked you pasta three times a day; then you wouldn't be having this big problem right now!*

Our true concerns were not accurately represented by our respective positions. Wayne's position was "Let's go eat Italian food tonight." Mary's position was "I don't feel like eating Italian food tonight." The underlying issues were not identified or spoken about in our foolishly escalating argument. Furthermore, our positions misrepresented certain important parts of our underlying interests.

Once we calmed downed and discussed this, we got to the most important points: Our respective underlying issues. Wayne's underlying issue was "I miss Mary. I wish that we could have a date tonight, go someplace quiet and relaxing, talk about our lives, connect with each other." Mary's underlying issue was quite simple: "I have indigestion. I don't feel like eating spicy food."

If either of us had been able to accurately identify and appropriately express our underlying issue, it is quite likely that we would have more quickly reached a satisfactory—and satisfying!—compromise. The conversation might have continued in this way:

Wayne: *I'm disappointed that you don't want to go out. I thought you'd be excited about having a "date" in the middle of the week. The weekend seems a long way away.*

Mary: *Wayne, I just don't feel like eating spicy food. I didn't say that I didn't want to have a "date" with you.*

Wayne: *Wait a minute. What are we talking about here? I don't really care what kind of food we eat; I want you, not the food! I just thought that the Italian restaurant would be a romantic place to go.*

Mary: *Well, I would love for us to spend the evening together. But I'm not going to be a very good date if I have indigestion. Why don't we stay home, put the kids to bed early, and talk about our life over a nice glass of Alka-Seltzer?*

A key to clarifying your underlying issues is to look forward, not back, during your discussions. As tensions escalate during conflict, we all tend to throw unfinished business into the pot of the current conversation. Wayne hinted at doing this with his "You never cook Italian food anymore" statement. Looking backward during an argument only serves to escalate defensiveness and conflict. Look forward. Talk about what you would like to see happen, not about past resentments. If you are harboring pain from a past hurt, that topic deserves a separate discussion. Don't try to resolve everything during one negotiation; doing so only muddies the water and makes it difficult to resolve anything.

In a nutshell, effective negotiation requires that you not get stuck in an angry posture that simply fuels further anger. Try to identify and communicate your own and the other person's underlying needs during conflict. In noninflammatory language, clarify your position and reflect an awareness of the other person's position.

- Don't criticize; apologize.
- Don't deny your anger; reframe it as concern about what is happening.
- Don't displace your anger from one person or situation onto another person or situation; deal directly with the person or situation that is bothering you.

g. Rehearse. How many complex skills have you mastered without practicing them? As with learning anything new, it is important to rehearse appropriate anger management skills. Practice how you plan to respond to specific, upcoming situations. Role play your reactions. Picture yourself responding in ways that are effective. For example, you might use these techniques to prepare for a scheduled follow-up to deal with a specific conflict.

- Specify what points you want to get across in the follow-up.
- Recall effective versus ineffective ways of dealing with conflict.
- Specify *how* you would like to behave as you are conveying these points.
- Then practice behaving in these ways.

Some of this practice should be behavioral—stand before a mirror and pretend that you are dealing with the person with whom you have scheduled the follow-up. As you rehearse, notice yourself from the perspectives outlined in the *Ways to Fuel Anger* table.

Next, relax and use mental imagery to see, hear, and feel yourself dealing effectively in this situation. Replay a positive mental image over and over again until you can comfortably imagine yourself dealing effectively with the situation.

Practicing in this way has an added benefit. Soon the skills that you develop while rehearsing for anticipated situations become habits that serve you well in the heat of unanticipated bouts of anger.

h. Take a Leap of Faith. Finally, we recommend that you take a leap of faith in your ability to learn to control your anger and to better manage conflict. In our experience, folks who have been labeled as having hot tempers often accept the label as though this is a given and unchangeable fact about them. Even if you do tend to flare quickly, it is possible—and important—to learn to surround this tendency with skills that allow you to maintain control of your reactions.

Final Words

Anger and conflict are two of the most prevalent by-products of our busy lives. Mismanaging either can damage relationships, lower the quality of life, and limit productivity. However, the skills required for effective management of anger and conflict are learnable—and well worth learning.

References

1. Sotile WM, Sotile MO. The angry physician, I: the temper-tantruming physician. *Physician Executive.* 1996;22:30-34.
2. Sotile WM, Sotile MO. The angry physician, II: managing yourself while managing others. *Physician Executive.* 1996;22: 39-42.
3. Karasek R. *Healthy Work: Stress, Productivity and the Restructuring of Working Life.* New York, NY: Basic Books; 1992.
4. Smith TW. Hostility and health: current status of a psychosomatic hypothesis. *Health Psychol.* 1992;11:139-150.
5. Smith TW, Anderson NB. Models of personality and disease: an interactional approach to Type A behavior and cardiovascular risk. *J Pers Soc Psychol.* 1986;50:1166-1173.

6. Williams RB, Williams VP. *Anger Kills: Seventeen Strategies for Controlling the Hostility That Can Harm Your Health.* New York, NY: Time Books; 1993:xiii.
7. Gottman J, Silver. *Seven Principles for Making Marriage Work.* New York: Crown Publishers; 1999.
8. Waitley D. *How to Handle Conflict and Manage Anger: Action Guide.* Niles, Ill: Nightingale-Conant Corp; 1995. As modified in: Sotile WM, Sotile MO. Conflict management, part 1: how to shape positive relationships in medical practices and hospitals. *Physician Executive.* 1999;25:57-61. Also see: Sotile WM, Sotile MO. Conflict management, part 2: how to shape positive relationships in medical practices and hospitals. *Physician Executive.* 1999;25:51-55.
9. Sotile WM. Anger and hostility: assessment and treatment strategies. In: Wenger N, Smith K, Froelicher E, Comoss P, eds. *Cardiac Rehabilitation: Guide to Procedures for the 21st Century.* New York, NY: Marcel Dekker; 1998.
10. Alan R: Anger management: a systemic program to reduce unwanted anger. In: *Proceedings of the Third National Conference of the Psychology of Health, Immunity and Disease.* Orlando, Fla: The National Institute for the Clinical Application of Behavioral Medicine; 1991.
11. Sotile WM. *Heart Illness and Intimacy: How Caring Relationships Aid Recovery.* Baltimore, Md: Johns Hopkins University Press; 1992.
12. Siegman AW, Anderson RA, Berger T: The angry voice: its effects on the experience of anger and cardiovascular reactivity. *Psychosom Med.* 1991;52:631-643.
13. Siegman AW: The role of hostility, neuroticism, and speech style in coronary artery disease. In: Siegman AW, Dembroski TM, eds. *In Search of Coronary-Prone Behavior* (65-89). Hillsdale, NJ: Erlbaum; 1989.
14. Adapted from: McKay M, Rogers PD, McKay J. *When Anger Hurts: Quieting the Storm Within.* Oakland, Calif: New Harbinger Publications, Inc; 1989.
15. Fisher R, Ury W. *Getting to Yes: Negotiating Agreement Without Giving In.* 2nd ed. New York, NY: Penguin Books; 1991.

Further Reading

For information on anger management:

Williams RB, Williams VP. *Anger Kills: Seventeen Strategies for Controlling the Hostility That Can Harm Your Health.* New York, NY: Time Books; 1993.

McKay M, Rogers PD, McKay J. *When Anger Hurts: Quieting the Storm Within.* Oakland, Calif: New Harbinger Publications, Inc; 1989.

Alan R: Anger management: a systemic program to reduce unwanted anger. In: *Proceedings of the Third National Conference of the Psychology of Health, Immunity and Disease;* Orlando, Fla: The National Institute for the Clinical Application of Behavioral Medicine; 1991.

Sotile WM. Anger and hostility: assessment and treatment strategies. In: Wenger N, Smith K, Froelicher E, Comoss P, eds. *Cardiac Rehabilitation: Guide to Procedures for the 21st Century.* New York, NY: Marcel Dekker; 1998.

For information on ways to foster a positive interpersonal culture in medical settings:

Sotile WM, Sotile MO. The angry physician, I: the temper-tantruming physician. *Physician Executive.* 1996;22:30-34.

Sotile WM, Sotile MO. The angry physician, II: managing yourself while managing others. *Physician Executive.* 1996;22:39-42.

Sotile WM, Sotile MO. Effective emotional management: keys to the balancing act facing contemporary administrators. *J Cardiovasc Manage.* 1996; 7:18-23.

Sotile WM, Sotile MO. Conflict management, part 1: how to shape positive relationships in medical practices and hospitals. *Physician Executive.* 1999;25:57-61.

Sotile WM, Sotile MO. Conflict management, part 2: how to shape positive relationships in medical practices and hospitals. *Physician Executive.* 1999;25:51-55.

For discussion of the psychodynamics of chronically angry people:

Matthews KA Woodall LK. Childhood origins of overt Type A behaviors and cardiovascular reactivity to behavioral stressors. *Ann Behav Med.* 1988;10:71-77.

Price V. *Type A Behavior Pattern: A Model for Research and Practice.* New York, NY: Academic Press; 1982.

For a discussion of the health effects of writing about upsetting feelings:

Pennebaker J. *Opening Up: The Healing Power of Confiding in Others.* New York, NY: Avon; 1991.

For information on the health risks of unchecked hostility:

Williams RB. Coronary-prone behaviors, hostility, and cardiovascular health: implications for behavioral and pharmacological interventions. In: Orth-Gomer K, Schneiderman N, eds. *Behavioral Medicine Approaches to Cardiovascular Disease Prevention.* Hillsdale, NJ: Lawrence Erlbaum Associates; 1996:161-168.

Smith TW. Hostility and health: current status of a psychosomatic hypothesis. *Health Psychol.* 1992;11:139-150.

For discussion of conflict negotiation:

Fisher R, Ury W. *Getting to Yes: Negotiating Agreement Without Giving In.* 2nd ed. New York, NY: Penguin Books; 1991.

Edelman J, Crain MB. *The Tao of Negotiation.* New York, NY: Harper Business; 1993.

Staver, M. *21 Ways to Diffuse Anger and Calm People Down.* Boulder, Colo: CareerTrack Pub; 1987.

Waitley D. *How to Handle Conflict and Manage Anger: Action Guide.* Niles, Ill: Nightingale-Conant Corp; 1995.

Chapter 15

Healthy High-Powered Relationships

A hero is someone who creates safe spaces for others.
        —Wayne & Mary Sotile

The keys to managing a high-powered medical life are maintaining positive relationships at work and intimacy at home. We have already described the various hurdles you must clear if your relationship is to survive. Here, we want to emphasize the flip side of the coin: the secrets of hundreds of medical couples we know who are using their skills and energy to create and maintain healthy relationships. A look at these remarkable couples will inspire you to keep winning in your marriage.

Pattern 8: Using Our Good Stuff to Make It Better

The *Using Our Good Stuff* medical couples share many characteristics with other patterns of medical marriage. These couples start their romances with their own versions of rose-colored glasses, intending for the relationship to be a place of refuge. Like others, they cooperate in gradually increasing the size and scope of their life together and fall into the same traps of fatigue, stress, and disillusionment that inevitably face all modern relationships. Just like everyone else, they, too, must periodically struggle through renegotiating their relationship contracts, and they find that life ends up being far more stressful and complex than anyone anticipated. The greatest pitfall for these exceptional couples is their humbling awareness that, no matter how much they love each other or how well they cooperate in running their lives and their relationship, they still do not prove to be the exception to the rules that apply to us all. The stresses of a demanding life periodically drain their energy and vitality.

However, unlike couples in the other patterns mentioned, these people do "use their good stuff." They dare to call on their high-powered, personality-based coping abilities to counter (rather than compound) their stress loads. More than anything, what distinguishes these couples from less healthy ones is their willingness to create and maintain loving cooperation and flexibility, especially during stress-filled passages in their years together. They refuse to settle into concretized patterns of imbalance among work, family, marriage, and self, or to lose sight of the effects they have on each other. They are committed to keeping the relationship an enduring, safe arena.

Exactly how is this done? With mature effort and acceptance of the fact that no one does it perfectly. No one can specify surefire guidelines for making anything as complicated as a marriage work smoothly. We won't insult you by offering any such cookbook formula. But we do want to describe various characteristics that we have noted in our study of medical couples who beat stress together:

- They manage the supercouple syndrome.
- They share responsibility respectfully and fairly.
- If they have children, they pay attention to parenting.
- They recognize situations and patterns that threaten their relationship and do something about them.
- They take responsibility for themselves.
- When needed, they seek help to manage stress and keep their marriage alive.
- They fight to keep romance alive in their marriage.
- They work together to create a "new normal" for medical marriages.

No couple perfectly embodies all eight of these characteristics. There are no perfect people, and there certainly are no perfect marriages. The *Using Our Good Stuff* medical couples try their best to assimilate these qualities, even though they fall short in some areas at various times.

Thriving Guideline 1: Manage Supercouple Syndrome

By now, it should be abundantly clear that we believe no medical couple is immune to supercouple syndrome: If you don't watch out, your busy life will compel you to cope in ways that hurt your relationship. Healthy medical couples work to manage both the impact of their respective coping styles on their relationship, and the impact of their relationship on each other's coping styles. In a nutshell, they follow the Do's and Dont's outlined below.

Helping Each Other to Do Your BEST

Do	Don't
• Acknowledge the relationship consequences of your respective coping styles	• Deny or lie
	• Pretend to be identical

Do	Don't
• Lower baseline levels of stress	• Live in chronic Hurry Sickness
• Use change strategies	• Stay numb
• Let some stuff slide	• Turn everything into an interpersonal issue
• Nurture self and spouse	• Blame or shame
• Bear through the awkwardness of changing	• Stay in a narrow comfort zone
• Push for healthiness	• Normalize drivenness
• Be specific regarding desired changes	• Let self be a target
• Practice pleasure	• Mess up to fit in
	• Organize life around blind ambition
	• Be vague
	• Work, work, work!

The key to beating stress together is to make a collaborative effort to prevent your high-powered coping styles from controlling your personal life. You must work to do so without defensiveness, blaming, or shaming. This requires that you communicate in ways that acknowledge your differences and, as much as is possible, help lower your respective baseline levels of stress. Doing so begins with an honest assessment of yourselves.

Use the following checklist to remind yourself and your partner of your stress symptoms. Use this information as a reminder to disrupt any tendency to ignore your stress "red flags," go numb to help endure your stress, and/or ignore the effects you have on those around you.

What Are Your Stress Symptoms?

Instructions: Check those symptoms and behaviors you typically experience, either before or after a stressful situation.

Physical Stress Symptoms: *When I am overstressed, my body reacts with* . . .

___Fast heartbeats	___Shallow breathing	___Tense shoulders/back
___Muscle twitching	___Heartburn	___Bowel problems
___Insomnia	___Fatigue	___Tearing eyes
___High blood pressure	___Perspiring	___Feeling flushed
___Dry mouth	___Headaches	___Backaches
___Jaw pain	___Skin problems	___Hives
___Excessive appetite	___Loss of appetite	___Other

Stress Emotions: *When I am overstressed, I tend to feel* . . .

___Sad	___Lonely	___Angry
___Anxious	___Disgusted	___Contemptuous
___Manic	___Energized	___Fearful
___Discouraged	___Helpless	___Shy
___Paralyzed	___Scattered	___Numbed
___Other_____		

Stress Thinking: *When I am overstressed, my thinking drifts toward . . .*

___Worrying	___Worst-case thinking	___Personalizing blame
___All-or-nothing thinking	___Selectively perceive negatives	___Difficulty focusing
___Difficulty concentrating	___Obsessive rumination	___Angry thoughts
___Thoughts of persecution	___Self-pitying thoughts	___Blaming others

___Other_____

Stress Behaviors: *When I am overstressed, I tend to . . .*

___Rush	___Overwork	___Drive aggressively
___Slow down	___Smoke	___Overuse alcohol or drugs
___Use illegal drugs	___Overeat	___Undereat
___Sleep excessively	___Have insomnia	___Exercise excessively
___Become sedentary	___Excessively use escapism	___Procrastinate

___Other_____

Interpersonal Behaviors: *When I am overstressed, my interpersonal style tends to be . . .*

___Argumentative	___Controlling	___Competitive
___Defensive	___Sarcastic	___Act bored
___Uncooperative	___Passive-aggressive	___Overly sensitive
___Unaffectionate	___Needy	___Unassertive or passive
___Aggressive	___Brusque	___Hurried

___Other_____

Next, use the following table to give each other feedback on your respective coping patterns.

Superachiever Scale: How Do You Compare?

Instructions: Use the following scale to rate yourselves on each of the characteristics listed.

1	2	3	4	5
never	sometimes	often	usually	always

	How often am I?	How often are you?
Time urgent		
Doing and thinking multiple things at once		
Impatient		
Perfectionistic		
Hostile/cynical		
Controlling		
Competitive		
Involved in work		
Hot-tempered		
Irritable		

We reiterate a point made earlier: It is not our intention to encourage you to label each other. This and the other exercises in this chapter are intended to help you self-appraise and lovingly discuss your similarities and differences. The point is to clarify ways that you can be helpful to each other in creating a more nurturing style of life.

The goal is to manage your stress reactions so that you can keep your relationship a pleasant and comfortable place where healthy pleasures are encouraged. Fortunately, these processes are complementary. For example, you can at once bolster your individual stress management capacity *and* enhance your relationship if you help each other slow down, at least in spurts. Living in chronic urgency perpetuates stress and kills caring connection. On the other hand, marital researchers and clinicians proclaim the good news that engaging in even brief (e.g., thirty-second to two-minute) spurts of caring interaction for a total of twenty to thirty minutes each day can significantly stress-proof your marriage.[1] Doing so serves two important purposes:

- It forces you to slow down and at least momentarily disrupt what otherwise will be your own escalating levels of tension and hurriedness.
- These brief moments of repeated, caring contact keep you reasonably connected with your loved ones, even through the busy times.

Having fun is another way to both counter stress and enhance your marriage. For couples with busy lives, the trick is to accept the fact that you must consciously make time and save energy to have fun. You must give up what family therapist Peter Fraenkel calls the "myth of spontaneity."[2] If not orchestrated, playful, romantic occasions tend to dwindle in inverse proportion to the rising stress in your life.

Here, beware of a mistake that many busy people make: They confuse *aversion relief* with true pleasure, perceiving the relief of working hard to accomplish a pressing task as having fun. The comments of one of our physician clients shows how this works.

M.O.S.: *So, how was your weekend?*
Client: *It was great. I had a great weekend.*
M.O.S.: *Did you? How so?*
Client: *Well, I just had a lot of fun. It was a good weekend.*
M.O.S.: *What was fun?*
Client: *Well, I wasn't on call, so I got up and had the weekend to myself. I finally got the time I needed to catch up.*
M.O.S.: *What do you mean?*
Client: *I woke up early and got my laundry started, then I got the grocery shopping done before the crowds converged on the supermarket. Then I finished up "my part" of one of my son's science projects—I love it when these teachers give seventh-graders science projects that it takes an M.D. to figure out.*

Did some more laundry while I tied up some loose ends from work: paperwork, correspondence, nothing heavy—just busywork that's been aggravating me and that I never find time to do.

M.O.S.: *What then?*

Client: *Well, my older daughter's car needed to have an oil change, so I arranged for that while she and I ran to the mall to shop for her school coat. She has been needing that coat for a month, but both of us hate shopping, so we've been putting off going. But we bit the bullet, fought the crowds, and got it done.*

M.O.S.: *And then?*

Client: *By the time we got home, everyone was getting hungry. I've been feeling bad about how often we eat out, so I decided to do that motherly thing. I threw together some dinner and began a pot of soup for us to eat throughout the week.*

M.O.S.: *What was the evening like?*

Client: *I caught up on some reading. I'm presenting a paper in two months at our national meeting, and I've been anxious about it. So I took Saturday evening to get a jump on the stack of journal articles that I've been accumulating since the paper got accepted. Nothing else was happening. My husband watched a ballgame on TV. My son had a friend spend the night. I just relaxed and read—in between trying to calm down my son and his rambunctious friend.*

M.O.S.: *Anything else?*

Client: *No, just relaxed and read ... finished up the laundry and the soup right before I went to bed at midnight.*

Does this sound like a fun weekend or what? While she obviously felt relieved that she had gotten all of these chores done, what this woman experienced was a far cry from pleasure. Her pleasure was akin to the relief you feel once a headache goes away: cessation of pain is not the same as pleasure!

Many high-powered people forget how to play. Researcher Ethel Roskies recommends the use of a pleasure log: a journal that records how much of your day is given to feelings of pleasure versus displeasure.[3]

The Pleasure Log*

1. Every hour on the hour, note your activity and how you feel in terms of "pleasure" or "displeasure." Then, note your feelings.

2. At the end of each day, add up the number of pleasures and displeasures.

Time	Activity	Pleasure	Displeasure	Feelings
6:00 AM				
7:00				
8:00				

Time	Activity	Pleasure	Displeasure	Feelings
9:00				
10:00				
11:00				
noon				
1:00 PM				
2:00				
3:00				
4:00				
5:00				
6:00				
7:00				
8:00				
9:00				
10:00				
11:00				
midnight				
TOTALS:				

*From Roskies E. *Stress Management for the Healthy Type A: Theory and Practice.* New York, NY: Guilford Press; 1987.

Thriving Guideline 2: Share Responsibility Respectfully and Fairly

You must share responsibilities. As any married couple knows, this does *not* mean a 50-50 division of labor in *every* area of your life. Rather, in general, you must work to maintain equity: The sum total of what each of you contributes to your life together needs to be roughly equivalent in value. And perhaps more importantly, each of you needs to *make note* of what the other gives and *regularly express appreciation* for all that your partner contributes to your life together.

The following is designed to help you give voice to ways that you appreciate each other.

The Marital Responsibilities Scale

Instructions:

1. Read through the following items and check who assumes responsibility for each of the aspects of marriage and family life that are listed. As you do so, bear two points in mind:

   a. The question is who assumes the responsibility for getting the work done in each area regardless of whether or not one of you actually does the work.

   b. Some couples share responsibility for a given area. Note if this is the case.

2. Using the following scale, record your estimate of the degree of comfort or discomfort the responsible person experiences in each area.

1	2	3	4	5
always easy to do	usually easy to do	benign	usually difficult to do	usually agonizing to do

3. Next, compute your respective total number of assumed responsibilities and total comfort/discomfort ratings.

4. Finally, divide your total comfort scores by the total number of areas of responsibility, as shown.

Responsibility	Assumed by		Comfort Level	
	Male:	Female:	Male: 1-5 *(see scale)*	Female: 1-5 *(see scale)*
Earns money				
Manages family budget				
Pays monthly bills				
Prepares income taxes				
Cleans house				
Nurtures family				
Remembers birthdays				
Takes charge of yard work				
Carpools or chauffeurs				
Arranges vacations				
Packs for vacations				
Grocery shops				
Clothes shops				
Gift shops				
Arranges social life				

Responsibility	Assumed by		Comfort Level	
	Male:	Female:	Male: 1-5 *(see scale)*	Female: 1-5 *(see scale)*
Monitors family's health				
Assumes role as religious leader				
Plays with children				
Disciplines children				
Keeps track of children's routines				
Maintains vehicles				
Calls repairmen				
Meets with repairmen				
Washes clothes				
Goes to the laundry				
Feeds family				
Cares for pets				
Takes out trash				
Clean up after meals				
Nurses the sick				
Takes care of elderly				
Other (specify as many as you like)				
Totals:	**Male**		**Female**	
Total comfort levels:				
Total number of areas of responsibility:				
Marital Responsibility (MR) Score:				
Male's total comfort level divided by male's number of respon-sibilities (MR Score)				
Female's total comfort level divided by female's number of respon-sibilities (MR Score)				

Interpretations of Marital Responsibilities Scale
Use the following guidelines as you discuss your responses.

1. Note discrepancies in your own and your partner's ratings.
   - When do you assume responsibility without your partner realizing it?
   - Where does your partner assume responsibility without your realizing it?
   - In which areas is your partner struggling more than you realized?
   - In which areas are you struggling more than you may have communicated?
   - In which areas is your partner actually struggling less than you assumed he or she was?
2. Discuss the following topics.
   - Which areas of your overall life are of most value to each of you, regardless of who assumes responsibility for these areas? How do you differ regarding your answers to this question?
   - Would you like to renegotiate the distribution of responsibilities within your relation-ship? If so, how so?
   - Which of the many areas of responsibility assumed by your partner do you most appreciate?

The point of this exercise is not to stir controversy in your marriage. Rather, we hope that it will help underscore how much each of you does· that is of value to the other person's life. Take time to elaborate on your appreciation of each other. Thriving couples don't take each other for granted; they notice and comment on each other's daily acts of heroism.

Thriving Guideline 3: Pay Attention to Your Parenting

We include this guideline at the risk of stating the obvious: Of course parents must parent together. But in many medical families, this is an underdiscussed topic. A thorough review of the medical literature indicates that amazingly little has been written about growing up in a medical family.

Perhaps this relative lack of attention to this topic reflects what we believe to be our culture's unfortunate malaise about the impact of marital dynamics on children. Careful family researchers have recently refuted the often-bantered-about notion that marital conflict is often worse for children than divorce. While no one disputes the fact that marital conflict can be damaging to children, contemporary researchers have demonstrated that the effects clearly become stronger when the parents are in fact divorced.[4] Recent surveys have found that, when children from broken homes become teenagers, they have two to three times more behavioral and psychological problems than do children from intact homes. Summarizing research in this area, imminent family researcher David Blankenhorn, Ph.D., president of the Institute for American Values, had this to say: "Youngsters from stable intact families have the strongest sense of well-being. Youngsters from single-parent families are the worst off, despite the fact that the divorce may have taken place ten years ago, and even after controlling for income."[5]

We offer a few cautionary concepts, based on our clinical experiences both with medical couples and with children of physicians.

First, pay attention to what your lifestyle is teaching your children. Don't make the mistake of only showing your children your pain—your fatigue, worry, stress, or criticism. Periodically take a break from being your children's teacher or monitor and simply spend time with them, showing them your playful and accepting side. And beware of the tendency of many superachiever parents to shame their children into developing driven, Type A coping styles as early as age five. Of course, all parents want our children to learn to be responsible people, but beware of conveying disapproval of a child being playful, "wasting time," or otherwise engaging in those activities at which most of us driven adults aspire to be better.

Second, creatively establish and protect family rituals. Here, we emphasize the need to be creative. The "dinner at 6:00 p.m." ritual of yesteryear is unrealistic for many families today. And being overly rigid about the exact form of a ritual defeats the point: Children benefit from family rituals that allow you, as a family, to change pace and spend time together, renewing your love and connection with each other. In this regard, a trip to the park, a family breakfast, or a fun night eating out at a favorite, family-friendly restaurant can be every bit as effective as the nightly dinnertime ritual.

Third, let your children know that you consider their issues and interests to be important. It's easy to forget how intimidating grown-up stressors—and, especially, a physician's work—can be to children. Show that you are interested in your children and that you admire them. Ask them to teach you what they know; brag about them openly in front of others. If you are not able to attend their special events, cooperate as parents in making big deals of what your children find to be important. Videotape the dance recital, ballgame, or class play, and then make a fun family production out of everyone celebrating the child's special moment.

This brings us to a third point: In our experience, father-physicians too frequently have limited intimate knowledge of who their children are. The "rule" that "Mom's responsible; Dad helps out" is still the prevailing theme around which most medical marriages operate, regardless of Mom's occupational status. Despite women's liberation, men's consciousness-raising, and the rising number of female professionals entering the workforce, it is still the mother who has the most involvement with the children. Accordingly, it is the mother who endures the most stress and enjoys the most intimate understanding of the kids.

In his book *Why Parents Disagree: How Women and Men Parent Differently and How We Can Work Together,*[6] psychologist Ron Taffel recommends that you periodically write down everything each of you does or thinks about in relation to your children during a given period of time, such as a weekend, weekday evening, or morning. Then compare lists. Taffel claims that even dads who are deemed *by their wives* to be very involved in fathering typically generate lists that pale in comparison to those of their wives. An example from Taffel:

> As Dennis's record showed, he *was* involved: calling home to see whether he should pick up anything, setting the dinner table, cleaning up around the house, checking on homework, reading and saying goodnight to the kids. Dennis, indeed, seemed to be a hands-on father—until Sabrina produced her list.
>
> Where Dennis had recorded a dozen tasks on a 3" x 5" index card, she (his wife) unfurled a six-foot scroll that covered almost 100 items. Reading them took the entire session. The following are only a sample: respond to kids badgering her about arrangements for the weekend and asking for permission about snacks; pack bags for sleepovers; pay bills; call other parents to set up play dates; braid her daughter's hair; make about 20 phone calls as

class mother; buy Christmas presents for the babysitter; do a load of washing; talk to her husband's mother (after he hands the phone to her); check the kids' homework; feed the cat; write thank-you notes for a recent birthday party.[7]

Now here is the point: The parent who participates in all of "the daily scut-work with kids," as Taffel calls it, will be the parent who is privy to those brief and fleeting moments when kids, operating *on their own schedule of when and how to communicate,* open up and tell you who they are. Only a person who spends time meandering with children will get to know them: what they fear, what they cherish, what's on their minds. It is these facts upon which intimacy is based. Children feel closest to people who know the *details* of their lives: who their friends are, what their favorite music is, who's gossiping about whom, which teachers they love and which they hate, whom they idolize, which older kids intimidate and which titillate them, when their next math test is, what grade they made on the last test, and so on.

Now consider the plight of the typical medical couple in which the father is a physician (regardless of whether or not the mother is a physician, too): Father leaves home before the children wake up. He comes home when each child is already in his or her own room, out, or on the phone. He interacts with the children in some way that is not based on any awareness of the details of their lives. For example:

Father: *Hey, Katherine. How are you?*
Child: *Fine.*
Father: *How was your day?*
Child: *Fine.*
Father: *What happened at school?*
Child: *Nothing.*
Father: *Do you have much homework?*
Child: *No.*
Father: *Well, what's going on?*
Child: *Nothing.*
Father: *Who are you talking with on the phone?*
Child: *A friend.*
Father: *Okay. Where's mom?*
Child: *In the kitchen.*

If this is the pattern, the physician-father will be relegated to the outside of his own family system, aware that his wife and children seem to be a family, while he is a busy, overstressed visitor. Taffel warns, "The pain men experience at being locked out of their children's lives and their dependence on their wives for entry is dangerous for families; it is one of the reasons fathers feel compelled to lecture, criticize or bully children."[8]

One physician whom we counseled for his temper outbursts responded to the above information with a tearful admission: "I know that I'm a 'hot reactor.' But that's not the only reason I get so angry at home. It's not just that the kids drive me crazy with all of their comings and goings and bickering and sassing their mother. It's that I'm not a part of it. I feel left out. In my own family, I feel left out. I look at them—bickering and laughing and horsing around with their mom—and I know that I'm not a part of that. I strike out trying to get in."

This same pattern can compromise your children's well-being, too.

Finally, a test: If you want to have psychologically healthy children, which of the following is the single best thing you can do?

- Build their self-esteem.
- Give them lots of hugging and cuddling.
- Provide firm, fair discipline.
- Make your spouse your equal partner and best friend.

Answer: The single best way to ensure having psychologically healthy children is to make your spouse your equal partner and best friend.

The Young Family Project at the Timberlawn Psychiatric Research Foundation in Dallas, Texas, followed couples for seven years in an effort to determine what characterizes healthy families. The data from this study show definite links between good marital dynamics and children's healthy development. If you want to raise healthy children, you must work out your *marital* issues regarding power, commitment, closeness, intimacy, and autonomy.[8]

Thriving medical couples who have children commit themselves to sharing both the joys and burdens of parenting. Even though one of them (typically the wife) functions as the primary parent, as couples these people do a great deal of tag-team parenting; they don't allow career- or gender-related issues to keep them from being active coparents. This means that the husband-fathers in these marriages face their gender-specific issues: they learn not to run from the anxiety, boredom, or sadness they might feel when they dare to father their children in ways in which they themselves may never have been fathered. With this sort of effort, couples are able to regularly create moments of family time in which the haze of their busy life clears and they are able to savor each other as partners in their ultimate creation—their children.

Thriving Guideline 4: Recognize High-Risk Situations and Patterns and Do Something About Them

As we stated earlier, stress-management experts propose that 80 percent of the stress we encounter can be anticipated and stress-management problems result when we lie about or deny—to ourselves or each other—what is coming up. A common characteristic among the many thriving medical couples whom we know is their honesty. They are realistic as they go about identifying the major factors that impact them or their marriage and family. They acknowledge that the challenges they face in managing themselves as a medical couple can only be mastered if they meet them head-on and with teamwork.

While there is no end to the possible challenges that you may face as a medical couple, we have noticed that thriving medical marriages are especially likely to proactively address several specific stressors. The following six points should be kept in mind as you decide what to do about high-risk situations and coping patterns.

1. Beware of High Risk Times. Research on physician divorce suggests that two stages of medical marriage carry special risks of promoting disillusionment. For those who marry during medical school or residency, the divorce statistics peak immediately following completion of training.

If you dodge this bullet (or if you marry later in life), statisticians warn, you should beware of the period approximately ten to fifteen years after entering practice. For those physicians who eventually divorce, the average length of marriage prior to separation is about twelve years; the average age at the time of divorce is forty-three years.[10,11]

If you recognize that disillusionment is a common occurrence during these stages of marriage, you are more likely to successfully anticipate (and not overreact to) tensions in your marriage. We certainly recommend that you *react*: with a redoubling of effort to correct what is wrong, not with a dash to divorce court. Better yet, we recommend that you do all that you can to bolster the strength of your marriage as you *approach* these times.

2. Be Realistic and Honest About Family Planning. One of the worst mistakes a medical couple can make is to pretend that the decision about whether or when to have children is solely up to the wife. It continues to amaze us how often medical couples, especially those consisting of a physician-husband and a nonphysician wife, make this mistake.

Be realistic about the fact that a new baby will create additional stress as well as new opportunities for you to deepen your bond with each other. Deal with the stress of the new arrival in a way that increases your trust in, intimacy with, and respect for each other, not in ways that will damage your relationship. The wounds that occur when a woman's husband is not there for her as she grapples with the decision to have a baby, goes through pregnancy and childbirth, or learns how to be a mother may never fully heal. We have heard countless bitter stories from wives about how physician-husbands abandoned them during such times:

Jeanie, wife of a pulmonologist: *"He left the decision about getting an abortion or having the baby up to me. I don't think he cared—he didn't care about me or what I was going through. I will never forgive him for that."*

Lucy, wife of a resident: *"What still makes me cry is the image of myself, a young woman who had never been through this before, alone and away from my family, having my baby with a nurse coaching me through it. I don't even remember the nurse's name, only her face and her voice. My husband was off sewing up other people in some emergency room across town. I know that we needed the money and that was why he was moonlighting. But I wish that he had been there with me, just that one night. That's all: just that one night."*

Christina, wife of Peter, a family-practice physician: *"I was so lonely until our first child was born. Then I got tired of being a 'single parent.' I talked with Peter about this when I found out that I was pregnant with our second baby, and he swore to me that he would change. I was like a new bride during that pregnancy; I felt that this baby was going to bring my husband back into my life and that we would once again be together, doing something that meant everything to me.*

"But that's not the way it went. Once the baby came, he worked more, was gone more, bullied me more, criticized more, and spoke to me less. I left him because I didn't like him anymore. He turned into someone I loathed."

Kathleen, wife of Charley, an obstetrician-gynecologist: *"Maybe he thought that he was being helpful by staying so detached and matter-of-fact throughout my delivery. I don't know. All I know is that I felt like I went through that entire labor and childbirth alone, with the help of 'medical personnel.' Unfortunately, Charley was just one of the 'medical personnel.' I wanted Charley, my husband, to be there instead."*

In contrast to these case vignettes, thriving couples have many different tales to tell about how they handled such critical times. They prepared for parenthood with lengthy, loving discussions about what life would be like when their babies arrived. They arranged their lives to be there for each other, emotionally and, when possible, physically. They strengthened their connection by responding compassionately to each other's experiences as they grappled with decisions and events surrounding pregnancy and childbirth.

In a related vein, women physicians in thriving marriages are supported in their efforts to plan for a good balance between career issues and creating and raising a family. This may mean delaying the timing of pregnancy until completion of training. Or, it might mean choosing a place of training or work based largely on the institution's policies and attitudes toward physician pregnancies, physician mothers, or job sharing with other women or men who may also want time to raise their families. Most importantly, women physicians struggling with such issues need the support of their husbands.

3. Counter Workaholism. Compared to nonprofessional workers, physicians work more hours, reap more fruits from their labors, and are more preoccupied with their work. They also tend to enjoy their work more than others.

It is not necessary to curb your interest and involvement in medicine in order to have a successful medical marriage. It *is* necessary to avoid workaholism, blindly committing to increasing the size and pace of your workload and ignoring symptoms of fatigue and distress or signals that your relationship is suffering from neglect. Nearly a quarter of a century ago, physician C. D. Chessick advised his colleagues to dare to create balance in their lives when he described the thriving physician as one who is "keeping up with and contributing to medicine, cultivating the mind through art and music and contemplation of life in terms of first principles, that is—what is true, what is good, what is valuable."[11]

While workaholism can drain the zest out of anyone, for physicians, it is epidemic. A survey of the stress-management techniques employed by 100 physicians (ninety males and ten females) found that only sixteen read for pleasure, attended theater or concert performances, or viewed television as a pastime. Only ten reported that they regularly took time off from work to relax. Only eleven of the physicians claimed that they took vacations exclusively for vacation's sake; fifteen indicated that they tried to combine "vacation" with professional meetings. The most common form of "relaxation" reported by the physicians in this survey was "working around the house."[12]

Of course, by now it should be clear that we believe that both spouses in a medical marriage are at risk of developing work addiction. How can you tell if this is happening to you? In *Work Addiction and Overdoing It: How to Slow Down and Take Care of Yourself*, author Bryan Robinson cautions that the following characteristics signal workaholism.[13]

Signs of Work Addiction

- Hurrying and staying busy
- Struggling with an excessive need to control
- Perfectionism
- Difficulty with relationships
- Work binges: Work highs lead to a work hangover, withdrawal, anxiety, and depression
- In advanced stages, work binges are concealed to avoid disapproval
- Difficulty relaxing and having fun
- Brownouts due to exhaustion and mental preoccupation with planning and work
- Impatience and irritability
- Self-inadequacy
- Self-neglect

Taking control of work addiction begins with an honest appraisal of your respective work habits. You can do this by discussing key points drawn from our modification of Robinson's *Work Addiction Risk Test,* originally published in our book, *Beat Stress Together: The BEST Way to a Passionate Marriage, A Healthy Family, and a Productive Life.* As you respond to the following scale, be sure to interpret *"work"* as applying to your life's work—that combination of obligations, roles, and responsibilities that you feel are part of your "job."

The Work Addiction Risk Test (WART): Couple's Form

Instructions: Use the following scale to rate how much each statement pertains to you and to your partner. Be sure to interpret "work" as that combination of obligations, roles, and responsibilities that you feel are part of your "job."

1	2	3	4	5
never true	sometimes true	often true	usually true	always true

Scores:

Mine	Yours	
		I prefer to do most things myself rather than ask for help.
		I get impatient when I have to wait for someone else or when something takes too long, like long slow-moving lines.
		I seem to be in a hurry and racing against the clock.
		I get irritated when I am interrupted while I am in the middle of something.
		I stay busy and keep many irons in the fire.
		I find myself doing two or three things at one time, such as eating lunch and writing a memo while talking on the phone.
		I overcommit myself by biting off more than I can chew.
		I feel guilty when I am not working on something.
		It is important that I see the concrete results of what I do.
		I am more interested in the final results of my work than in the process.
		Things just never seem to move fast enough or get done fast enough for me.
		I lose my temper when things don't go my way or work out to suit me.
		I sometimes ask the same question, without realizing it, after I've already been given the answer.
		I spend a lot of time mentally planning and thinking about future events while tuning out the here and now.
		I find myself continuing to work after my coworkers have called it quits.
		I get angry when people don't meet my standards of perfection.
		I get upset when I am in situations in which I cannot be in control.

Mine	Yours	
		I tend to put myself under pressure with self-imposed deadlines.
		It is hard for me to relax when I'm not working.
		I spend more time working than socializing with friends, on hobbies, or on leisure activities.
		I dive into projects to get a head start before all the phases have been finalized.
		I get upset with myself for making even the smallest mistake.
		I put more thought, time, and energy into my work than I do into my relationships with my partner, friends, and loved ones.
		I forget, ignore, or minimize important family celebrations such as birthdays, reunions, anniversaries, or holidays.
		I make important decisions before I have all the facts and have a chance to think them through thoroughly.

Compute your respective total scores.

Totals: Mine _____   **Yours** _____

Scoring

25-49 = You are not work addicted.

50-69 = You are mildly work addicted.

70-100 = You are highly work addicted.

*Reprinted with permission from: Sotile WM, Sotile MO. *Beat Stress Together: The BEST Way to a Passionate Marriage, A Healthy Family, and a Productive Life.* New York, NY: John Wiley & Sons, Inc; 1999.

Use the following guidelines to assure that your discussion is helpful, not critical of each other:

- Note how you each define your own and each other's "work."
- Note where you agree and disagree in self- and other-descriptions.
- Note changes in perceptions of each other: Have you changed in ways that your partner is not recognizing?
- What are small changes in your own and in your partner's work style or work orientation that might make a difference in the quality of your day-to-day life together?

It has been shown that, short of extraordinary lengths, long work hours are not associated with poor quality in medical marriages. Many physicians who regularly work sixty-five to seventy-five hours per week report very satisfying marriages and thriving careers.

We are *not* encouraging you to work that many hours per week, or saying that if you work even longer hours, your marriage is doomed. We simply make this point: What *does* determine overall quality of life for physicians, as with high-powered men and women in any other profession, is the extent to which they give and receive emotional support and engage in appropriate management of their own physical and emotional health.

To avoid workaholism, those proverbial "thriving medical couples" help each other to regularly pause, clarify their values, and honestly assess whether their behaviors are in harmony with their inner needs as individuals *and* as couples. Even if working hard is a strong value (and it typically is for medical couples), it is important to remind each other of the value of enjoying, not just struggling through, life. Based on such feedback and self-observation, thriving couples make adjustments that move them away from workaholism.

4. Use Your Resources to Save Your Time and Energy. Thriving medical couples acknowledge that while there may be time to "do it all" (or most of it) in the course of a lifetime, you can't be and do all things during any single stage of life. You have to choose which aspects of your life you will manage and which you will delegate. As one of our physician-patients put it:

I wish that I had time and energy to do my own yard work and to do the handyman stuff around my own house. That's what my father and all of the elders in my family did. Being self-sufficient was an important part of their identity; it has been a masculine family legacy. 'We Cromwells take care of ourselves.' I cringe whenever I call a repairman or pay that landscaping service to cut my grass. My ancestors are rolling over in their graves.

I also want to be more involved in my community—to give something back. Before medical school, I was a political leader in student government and a volunteer. I was also involved in state politics. I believe in getting involved.

Now I just don't take the time to do this stuff. There aren't enough hours in the week. But even though I'm not directly involved in these areas, I pay attention and contribute. I know what needs to be done to keep my house a place that I'm proud of, and I hire the best people to get the job done. I pay attention to local and state-level politics, and I contribute money and write letters and an occasional editorial.

Someday, when the kids are grown, I'll get more involved. But for now, my plate is full enough with other things that also matter to me.

In this same spirit, thriving medical couples use their resources to create a support system that simplifies their lives and helps them to beat stress together. They hire live-in help, people to do manual labor or household chores, cooks, professional shoppers, secretaries, and assistants (we are not referring to stereotypical "jet-setters" who do all of the above and then farm out their kids and take separate vacations).

Thriving medical couples do all of the above to buy time and energy to spend *with each other and their family*. As a physician friend of ours explained:

My husband and I earn $350,000 a year. We know that this is far more than most families have to live on. But we also know that our work and what it does to us causes more stress than most families have to live with. To compensate, we arrange our life so that when we're not working, we are available to our family and each other.

This has been a harder decision than it might seem. For example, we periodically "discover" that we could "afford" a second home or a house that is twice the size of the one we live in. It's been hard to resist the temptation to head down the same road that most of our friends have taken.

But we know that to do so would take most of our income. We've decided to stay put and use our financial cushion to buy quality in our life. Thank goodness we agree on this, because if not, I suspect we would have bought our piece of the mortgage pie or worn each other out fighting about it.

Given the inherent conflict between work versus domestic pull for physician-mothers, it is essential that they use their resources to arrange for the best child care available. But if good child care is readily available, it is easy to drift into workaholism. The point is to use your resources to buy time and energy for your personal life, not work.

5. Create Islands of Time During Which You Do Just One Thing at a Time. Hurry Sickness inspires us all to do and think more than one thing at once. While this talent is necessary and adaptive in many areas of life, it works against controlling stress and connecting with loved ones. Medical couples who thrive regularly take time to tune into each other and to be alone with and attentive to each of their children. Creating these islands of time builds relationships and keeps them alive.

The teenage daughter of two physicians spoke of the consequences of not following this advice:

Yeah, I get along with my dad okay.

No, I wouldn't say that we're really close; but we get along okay. . . .

We're not close because he doesn't really know me. I mean, he knows me, of course. God, he knows everything I do wrong; sometimes before I even do it!

But I don't know, it just seems that he's not very tuned in. You know what I mean? For example, my best friend is Lee. His dad's a physician, too; he knows what I'm talking about. Like, when I was a kid, I used to go to my dad's office after school to do my homework. This was right after he became the chairman or something. Anyway, what I remember is that if my mom had to finish her rounds, I went to my dad's office. I loved that office! He had the nicest office of any of the faculty. His desk and furniture were all wood, rich and important looking. I remember how it smelled in there.

Well, anyway, my dad would be in and out, talking on the phone or to other physicians, doing paperwork, all sorts of things. I used to love it when he was at his desk and I was doing my homework. We would chitchat while he was doing his work. He would ask things like "What are you doing?" and I'd say, "Homework." And he'd say, "That's nice." Then he'd keep on doing his work.

I love being around my dad because he's always so calm. But it's still sorta like when I was a kid in that office doing homework. I don't know, I wish I knew how to talk to him or something. If I try to tell him about myself, he seems in a hurry or something. Or we get interrupted, or I seem to be bothering him because he's so busy, I guess. Sometimes he just gives me one of his "fatherly advice" lectures.

That's what my friend Lee and I were talking about, those "fatherly advice" lectures.

A cartoon by Bill Keene once depicted a small child tugging at the sleeve of her father as he sat in his wing-backed chair, intent on reading the newspaper. The caption read: "But you have to listen with your *eyes*, Daddy, not just with your *ears*."

6. Be Honest if You Are at Risk of Burnout. Studies indicate that those physicians who enter the profession suffering from fundamental insecurity and a sense of inadequacy, low self-esteem, dependency, passivity, social anxiety, and tendencies toward obsessive worrying and depression are at risk of having the stresses of medical life drive them into serious adjustment problems. In addition, the "narcissistically vulnerable," those who have not historically received their fair share of unconditional love and attention, are at particular risk of struggling in close relationships even if their medical careers go well.

The warning signs of burnout are quite clear. You know you may be close to burnout if:

- You find yourself tiring ever sooner in the course of the week than you used to, saying something like, "I can't believe it's only Tuesday! It seems like the week should be ending by now."
- For no medical reason, you become more forgetful than usual.
- You are too busy to do routine tasks.
- You become resentful of routine demands made by others or by your work or family life.
- You are working hard but feeling like you are accomplishing less.
- You frequently end your days with a sense of sad exasperation about not having enough . . . time, accomplishments, success, acknowledgment, thanks, and so on.
- Your life and your work feel less satisfying.

- Typically pleasant events become chores (e.g., holiday, family outings, your office party).
- You have an increasing sense of depersonalization when interacting with others.

We have worked with a number of physicians who have suffered from these "warning signs" but did *not* become casualties. On the contrary, they created their fair share of fulfillment, happiness, and success, both professionally and personally. How did these people manage to rise above their inherent tendencies to burnout? How did they avoid crises in their marriage and family relationships? They had the sense and courage to commit themselves to changing, and, when necessary, to seek help.

Thriving Guideline 5: Heal Thyselves

By working together, you can create and maintain nurturing and affirming life "territories" and, within these territories, manage yourselves personally, professionally, and as a couple. Thriving medical couples (when possible) choose their situations wisely. They select specialties and work environments that allow for reasonable comfort and participation in their personal lives.

They also monitor their lives, especially during stressful times. Rather than simply going numb and soldiering on, they recognize particularly high-stress times and take care to be extra nurturing of themselves and of each other. They make concessions during the childbearing or child-rearing years. When faced with inevitable absences from each other due to career demands, they nurture themselves rather than simply suffering through.

No medical marriage can be healthy without a healthy physician. As George Vaillant put it, "The care of other people rather than of oneself is a superb form of adaptation—but only if the self is also cared for."[14] One of our patients, a physician's spouse, said,

Why should I listen to what my husband says about how to make our marriage better? He can't even take care of himself, for God's sake! He doesn't eat healthily. He's a stressed-out wreck half the time. He's even convinced himself that he 'really' needs only four hours of sleep a night. Frankly, I'm afraid to follow his 'advice.' I don't want to end up like him!

Thriving medical couples embrace principles drawn from the growing literature on ways that physicians can manage the stresses that come with the medical profession:

- **Claim your time.** Pause repeatedly throughout the day, even if for only a moment, before addressing your next task.
- **Make time for your loved ones**. When possible, limit on-call, weekend, and evening work. Take many minivacations. Set reasonable limits on the extent to which you are available to patients and colleagues.

- **Practice positive relationship skills** like listening, attentiveness, and reflecting on what others say. Be supportive. Show trust in selected people by sharing your feelings with them. Discuss with others your personal philosophies concerning creating a balance in your life.
- **Manage your outlook** by using reframing and relabeling techniques. For example:
- **Learn to use humor.**
- **View setbacks as learning experiences,** changes as challenges, stressful times as necessary steps toward desired goals, and vulnerable feelings as powerful resources rather than weaknesses to be overcome.
- **Remind yourself that death is not always a villain;** it is sometimes a friend that alleviates suffering.
- **Remember that uncertainty is often due to the nature of medical science,** not to your personal limitations.
- **Hear demands of patients as cries for help.**
- **When appropriate, remember to surrender.** Accept things that are beyond your control and use faith in some higher power to allow you to accept the limits of your power to control outcomes.
- **Allow yourself to grieve** the personal and professional losses that come your way. Acknowledge the deaths of patients who matter to you.
- **Seek out experiences that help you grow in healthy directions:** continuing education, keeping a personal journal, counseling, meditating, practicing yoga, religion, and so on.
- **View any unhealthy behavior patterns** or painful emotions, such as feelings of isolation or depression, as signals of a need to change.
- **Learn to be physically, emotionally, and spiritually nurturing** of yourself. Visit your physician, dentist, and counselor regularly. Take care of yourself through regular exercise, relaxation, prayer, proper nutrition, and limited use of alcohol, caffeine, and other drugs.

Thriving Guideline 6: Get Professional Help If You Need It

A common misconception is that physicians are too proud or stubborn to seek help even when it is painfully apparent that they need it. In truth, large percentages of M.D.s *do* get psychological help, but they usually wait until their problems are sufficiently severe. The reasons for the delay are not as predictable as you might think.

Sometimes physicians delay seeking help for themselves *and* sabotage their loved one's attempts at getting help because they have bought into the immature, grandiose notion that their identity is dependent on maintaining a "no problems" façade. We have worked with physically abused wives of physicians who have insisted on sneaking into our offices out of fear that their husbands' reputations will be tarnished if anyone finds out their "secret."

We have also worked with physicians who had alcohol or drug problems and feared that their professional reputations would be ruined if they sought help to become clean and sober. More than any other class of substance abusers we have worked with, physicians believe that the world will be rejecting and unsupportive if they admit their illness.

In one way or another, a delay in seeking help is often due to both partners in a medical marriage believing in a neurotic form of health: "If we keep up a frenetic enough pace and deny that any problems exist, this must mean that we are healthy."

In the sage words of physician Perry Ottenberg: "The sickest form of health is holding on to the pious belief in one's own invincibility when one is failing."[15]

Of course, such denial requires cooperation. Many physicians do not feel *entitled* to have problems or seek help, even though they know they need it. They do not live in denial but in pain that comes with passively accepting the role that they have been assigned in their families, practices, and culture. They have been "told" that they are supposed to be the paragons of health and hardiness, and they try to obey the injunction.

In other words, we find that the "let's not admit this, I'll be embarrassed" ethic can come not only from a driven, narcissistic physician, but also from an insecure family member or colleague who narcissistically acts as though the physician's admission of his humanness in some way tarnishes his or her own fragile halo. Pioneering researcher George Vaillant and colleagues cautioned that most physicians view distress in their lives with the attitude, "There is a lot wrong with me, but I will not inconvenience anyone else." These words still ring true.

We recommend that you place a sign over your back door that says "No Superpeople Live Here." As one of our physician clients explained:

> *It's a nice reminder that it's not only okay, it's expected that we will carry into our families our most human parts. Rather than leave our vulnerabilities and our sense of humor out in the garage, we want to leave that 'I'm the physician' armor in the trunks of our cars, ready to wear when we need it but aware that we don't need it when we are home.*

When the ethic in your marriage is that you are two good and imperfect people who are trying your best to manage your life, your relationship becomes a place to grow and struggle. When people in such relationships need help, they get it, and they cooperate with each other in the process.

In truth, physicians are especially likely to seek help if they think that their marriage is in trouble. In a study of 273 Alabama physicians[16] (94 percent were male, 77 percent were married, and their average age was forty-nine), 37 percent acknowledged having had problems, and 73 percent sought professional therapy (56 percent from a psychiatrist and 41 percent from a clinical psychologist). Furthermore, of those who sought help, 71 percent did so for marital problems, while another 32 percent sought help for the behavioral problems of their children. Another study of 747 physicians in Texas[17] found that, of those who complained of high levels of stress (a total of 173), 20 percent were actively involved in psychotherapy, while 34 percent were involved in marital therapy.

While a growing number of researchers suggest that, as a group, physicians who need it are quite responsive to marital therapy, it also seems that certain attitudes that cause problems in a physician's marriage can taint the therapeutic experience.

Managing Your Counseling

Any notion that the therapist will automatically align more with the physician-patient than the nonphysician-spouse has to be addressed. We have already described the tragic problem of a naive therapist's being co-opted by a defensive physician-spouse into discounting legitimate relationship issues by agreeing to diagnose the other spouse—rather than the marriage—as the patient.

In our experience, an equally likely scenario is the obsessive physician fearing that the marital therapist will automatically align with the nonphysician-spouse. The physician-patient sees the therapist as his or her competitor: The physician feels one-down as an "effective communicator with the opposite sex," a role that the therapist is supposedly expert in. This perceived competition can stir the physician's defensive need to prove his or her own competence by denying problems.

Finally, if it is to help, marital counseling cannot become a microcosm of one of the most prevalent problems in the medical marriage: the busy couple using professional responsibilities to dodge marital issues. When this happens, one or both members of the couple miss, cancel, or arrive late at appointments and in a state of exhaustion and hurriedness, always due to work demands. Counseling sessions are interrupted by beepers or emergency calls that are channeled into the session. In these ways, the marriage and family problems continue to be rationalized, neglected, or ignored.

Objectively, physicians' work does strain their personal lives, often stripping them of full control of their time. But a medical couple's management of these issues is often diagnostic of the state of their union—and prognostic of what is likely to happen in their marriage. Our clients have included medical students who had no say in determining their class or clinical schedules and private practitioners or senior-level medical administrators who were capable of scheduling appointments in any manner they desired. One overriding fact remains: If you are committed to getting help, you will find a way. You will either find a therapist whose schedule matches yours or change your schedules to match that of a therapist of your choosing.

Thriving Guideline 7: Fight to Keep Romance Alive in Your Marriage

In tangible ways, thriving medical couples fuel their romance. They embrace the characteristics of what could be called a formula for intimacy:

For a relationship to *work*, you need *communication*. But you need to balance problem-solving with *fun* and *cherishing*. *Trust* is essential, and it is created with *fairness* and *commitment*. By giving each other *permission to be complete persons* and by *forgiving* yourselves and each other for your imperfections, you can remain in love as you create a life together.[18]

We begin our counseling of medical couples with the challenge to create contexts that give three things a chance: your friendship, your communication, and your romance. Many of the tools and strategies that we have already outlined can improve your friendship and your communication. Here, we focus on ways to enhance your romance.

Start by accepting the truth: Fever-pitch romances only come in the form of a new relationship, particularly one that is fraught with a little drama or intrigue. Even the most passionate of couples tend to "cool" as the years progress.

But this does not mean that you should settle for being "bored and boring." In our opinion, the bane to romance in most relationships is not familiarity; it's laziness. We advise couples to continue to be mindful of the need to treat each other in that "boyfriend-girlfriend" way that originally lead to their falling in love. This message has many translations:

- **Continue to get to know each other.** Every week, learn something new about your spouse. Question and listen to each other. Notice each other. If you are not regularly learning something new about each other, you are not paying close enough attention.
- **Take a night off each week** to meander with each other. Use the following guidelines to structure these "dates": no working; no worrying; no washing the dishes; no discussing problems. Remind yourselves that you have worked harder than the vast majority of the people in the history of the human race, you certainly can afford to take a little recess!
- **At least once each month,** mark off a twelve- to forty-eight-hour period of time that will be protected as relationship time. If possible, use your resources (including your money, friends, and/or relatives) to free you up for a day or weekend escape together. This is a time to renew your nurturing, affectionate attention to each other. It may

take some getting used to, but bearing through the awkwardness is well worth the benefits that will come to your marriage.

- **Give each other personal surprises,** even years after the honeymoon is supposedly over.
- **Remember to be open, playful, and flexible in your sexual relationship,** even though the stresses and demands of your life (and aging) may change your sexual patterns. Research with couples under the age of sixty has clearly shown that frequency of sexual relations does not correlate with subjectively determined levels of satisfaction with one's sex life.[19] The crucial determiner is the couple's level of comfort discussing their sexual relationship with each other. Don't just do it; talk about it!
- **Acknowledge the grains of truth** in the other person's perceptions or opinions, even when dealing with your differences. We trust people who validate our perceptions even if they disagree with us. Show that you value each other.
- **Reaffirm your permission and encouragement to grow as individuals** as you go through periods of contract renegotiation in your marriage. Remember that marriage is about helping each other become complete, not a demand that both of you remain the same. Romance blossoms in relationships that free the individuals to be fully expressive of their respective selves. Strive to make your relationship a part of the solution, not a part of the problem.
- **Apologize and empathize.** No one escapes the need to "grow up" in the course of a marriage. Even though each of you is doing the best you can to cope with your complex life, inevitably you will make mistakes. In a spirit that says, "I am sorry that I didn't know better or didn't choose differently," apologize and empathize. Apologize for the pains that your struggles have caused your partner. Empathize with your partner's experience in the life you have worked together to create. And then forgive—yourself for your own shortcomings, and each other for having had to "grow up" in the course of this relationship.
- **Cherish each other.** Say nice things to each other and about each other when you are alone and in front of other people. When the person who knows you best says, "I know you, warts and all, and I still admire, love, respect, and want *you*," it touches your heart.

We challenge you to put aside any lies that you might tell yourself, such as: "All that love and romance business does not *really* happen in a real-life marriage." If you believe this, you are wrong. This is the hollow, self-centered mantra of a person who is unwilling to do what it takes to keep marriage alive. When you dare to look, proof of lifetime romance is all around you.

The forty-four-year marriage of the late actor Jimmy Stewart and his wife, Gloria, was a case in point. Gloria's 1994 obituary contained excerpts from an article in which a longtime friend talked about the special relationship the Stewarts enjoyed:

> To Jimmy, Gloria can do no wrong. She'll walk into a room and he will say, "You look wonderful tonight. What a wonderful dress." Gloria will respond, "Jimmy, I've worn it 10 times." Jimmy will respond, "You look beautiful." Even now, when she comes in from the garden in a T-shirt and jeans, he'll say, "You look better than anyone I've ever seen."[20]

We dare you to cherish each other in this way and see what happens to your romance.

- **Be generous and be gracious.** In our experience, high-intimacy couples are truly heroic; not in terms of doing extraordinary feats, but in our definition of the term: We believe that a *hero is someone who creates safe spaces for others.* How do they do this? With generosity and graciousness.

Romance grows when you generously present your partner the "gifts" that matter most to help him or her to feel safe, special, and loved. These gifts might take the form of special acts of attention or words of praise. For some, the greatest gift is your tolerance: of their passion for work or for your children; or of their need to attend to their aging parents. And remember to respond graciously to the gifts that your partner offers you, even if their offering was not your first choice. Few things are more hurtful than an ungracious response to a generously offered gift.

Thriving Guideline 8: Work Together to Create a "New Normal" for Medical Marriages

Medical couples who thrive refuse to accept outdated marriage-killer ethics that have pervaded their world for decades. They seem eager to help others do the same. This does not mean that they proselytize, but they are supportive of others' efforts to find balance in their lives. Rather than participating in any "conspiracy of silence," such couples speak the truth about the joys and struggles that come with a life in medicine—both to physicians and to their loved ones. In so doing, they validate and affirm each other.

More and more young medical couples are making career decisions by mutual consent rather than in blind deference to the male physician's career demands or preferences. For example, a recent survey of 245 fourth-year medical students in Toronto found that increasing numbers of residents consider training conditions like the availability of part-time work and parental leave in selecting a specialty.[21] In addition, increasing numbers of physicians are taking their spouses' needs into consideration in choosing residency placement and specialties, and both male and female physician graduates are voicing a desire for more flexibility in work arrangements. Nearly three fourths of young women physicians in Britain indicate that they would like to work part-time when their children are young,[22] and, worldwide, calls have been issued for more flexible training schedules and for job-sharing opportunities.[23]

Creative medical institutions and practices are responding to these influences. For example, at Colorado Permanente, 46 percent of women physicians work less than full time, as do 7.5 percent of male physicians.[24] A Seattle-based HMO, Group Health Cooperative, has a long history of job sharing, a policy that is officially encouraged by Britain's National Health system. In addition, examples of creative arrangements for flextime—the ability to group work hours into fewer than five-day weeks, thereby allowing for more work-free days per month—are growing in the literature. The effects of such policies on physician well-being and medical economics remain to be systematically evaluated.

Recent surveys of the personal lives of physicians are suggesting that, compared to prior generations, contemporary physicians are creating time to experience greater levels of personal, marital, and family pleasures in their day-to-day lives.[25] In the aforementioned study of 200 surgeon-spouse pairs, both the physicians and their spouses independently indicated that, while life certainly is stressful, they still spend an average of sixty-four to sixty-seven minutes each day in conversation with each other. Furthermore, these surgeons indicated that in a typical week they spend an average of 1.8 evenings devoted to activities with their children and approximately one evening per week exclusively with their spouses. These physicians took an average of 14.5 vacation days with their families annually and an additional 9.5 days with their spouses. Not surprisingly, those surveyed rated their marriages and careers gratifying or extremely gratifying.[25]

Modern-day physicians also realize their need for support. A survey of fifty-seven women and 147 men practicing medicine for one to four years noted that "80 percent of women and men physicians reported that there was someone other than their spouse or romantic partner whom they could turn to 'at any time' when they experienced problems."[26]

These people who fight for the right to live in healthy ways are also spearheading much-needed institutional-level changes in medicine. They support such humane, nonsexist institutional policies as part-time residency programs, generous leaves of absence for childbearing *and* child rearing, paternal as well as maternal and family leave, and retraining programs that would permit parents to return to the mainstream of medicine after a leave of absence. They also are resonating with the call delivered in a recent *JAMA* article[27] that highlighted the need to expand medical training to include courses on self-care, stress management, and strategies for juggling personal and professional responsibilities.

We add to this call the need to afford physicians *and their loved ones* opportunities to receive interpersonal skill training, both during medical training and in continuing educational programs.

These institutional-level changes are slow in coming. But at least the issues are being raised. And these efforts *are* paying off. Sanctions on the extent to which residents can be worked are being implemented worldwide. Britain's experiment with decreasing contract hours of hospital physicians to a maximum of seventy-two hours per week is now being modified to further lighten workloads for physicians-in-training. Currently, more than 75 percent of medical schools incorporate formal maternity leave policies for medical residents, a figure that is up from less than 50 percent of training institutions as recently as the late 1980s.[28]

Proposals that are being considered or implemented in various institutions include enforced periods during which physicians are not available for clinical activities, mandated complete use of vacation allotments, rotation of unpleasant administrative chores in academic medical departments, and explicit inclusion of medical families in institutional social activities; also, stress management and issues relevant to medical marriages and spouses of physicians are being addressed at major medical meetings.

Our own professional experiences are a testament to emerging changes. In recent years, we have been invited to speak on managing the stresses of medical practice and marriage and family life to literally hundreds of gatherings of medical professionals and their loved ones. These invitations have ranged from grand-rounds presentations at hospitals to banquets staged by state and regional medical society alliances and national meetings of prestigious medical organizations (e.g., the American College of Physicians and Surgeons; the American Urological Association; the American Association of Orthopaedic Surgeons; the American Society of Plastic and Reconstructive Surgery; and the American Society for Anesthesiologists).

In addition, progressive departments of mainstream medical specialties (such as the Department of Anesthesia at the University of Michigan Medical School in Ann Arbor and the Department of Orthopaedic Surgery at the Massachusetts General Hospital and Harvard Medical School) have invited us to be visiting professors—certainly not due to anything we know about their area of medical specialization, but out of concern for the most important common denominator in medicine: the people involved in the practice of the profession.

More than ever, physicians and their loved ones are using their considerable talents and resources to ensure their *own* health. Such efforts not only create greater personal satisfaction—they also help today's physicians keep their professional motivation and productivity flowing.

Conclusion

Is making a medical marriage work really worth all this effort?

Are the potential benefits from working to beat stress together worth the pain that comes from stretching your skills, insights, and typical ways of interacting?

We believe that the answer to this question is unequivocally "Yes!" Nothing feels worse than not getting along with one's mate, and few things feel as good as marital harmony.

People who live in supportive, loving relationships do indeed thrive, not just survive. They get sick less often and, if they do get sick, they tend to recover more fully. Whether we are studying specific illnesses, such as cancer or heart disease, or examining the effects of stress-filled, high-powered lives, we predict that the next two decades will definitively show that increasing intimacy in your life may be your most potent way to ensure health, productivity, and happiness. Getting along with each other is more than just improving the cosmetics of your life. Keeping your marriage vital may be your most powerful defense against the adverse effects of the stresses that come with a medical life.

Be heroes for each other. Do all that you can to make your marriage work. The rewards will far outweigh the effort.

References

1. Fraenkel P. Time and couples, part II: the sixty-second pleasure point. In: Nelson TS, Trepper TS, eds. *101 More Interventions in Family Therapy*. New York, NY: The Haworth Press; 1998:145-149.

2. Fraenkel P. Time and rhythm in couples. *Fam Process*. 1994;33(March):37-51.

3. Roskies E. *Stress Management for the Healthy Type A: Theory and Practice*. New York, NY: Guilford Press; 1987:206.

4. Spruijt E, de Goede MJ. Transitions in family structure and adolescent well-being. *Adolescence*. 1997;32:897-991.

5. Blankenhorn D. *Propositions: A Letter of Ideas and Findings*. New York, NY: Institute for American Values; 1999;4:1-12.

6. Tafell R. *Why Parents Disagree: How Women and Men Parent Differently and How We Can Work Together*. New York, NY: William Morrow; 1994.

7. From: Taffel R. The power of two. *Fam Ther Networker*. September/October 1994:47.

8. Lewis JM. The transition to parenthood, I: the rating of prenatal marital competence. *Fam Process*. 1988;27:149-165.

9. Eisenberg H, Kauffman HH, eds. Your family life: putting it all together. *Med Economics*. 1973;April (special issue): .

10. Segraves K, Segraves RT. When the physician's marriage is in trouble. *Med Aspects Hum Sexuality*. June 1987:48-159.

11. Chessick CD. On the quality of the physician's life. *Ill Med J*. 1969/70:136-174.

12. Krakowski AJ. Stress and the practice of medicine: the myth and the reality. *J Psychosom Res*. 1982;26:91-98.

13. Robinson B. *Chained to the Desk: A Guidebook for Workaholics, Their Partners and Children and the Clinicians Who Treat Them*. New York, NY: New York University Press; 1997.
14. Vaillant GE, Sobowale NC, McArthur C. Some psychologic vulnerabilities of physicians. *N Engl J Med*. 1972;287:372-375.
15. Ottenberg P. The physician's disease: success and work addiction. *Psychiatr Opin*. 1975;12:6-11.
16. Snider HS, Storm CL. A study of physicians as clients. *Fam Therapy*. 1989;16:69-78.
17. Lewis JM, Barnhart FD, Howard BL, Carson DI, Nace EP. Work stress in the lives of physicians. *Tex Med*. 1993;89:62-67.
18. Sotile WM. *Heart Illness and Intimacy: How Caring Relationships Aid Recovery*. Baltimore, Md: Johns Hopkins University Press; 1992:85.
19. Laumann EO, Michael RT, Gagnon JH, Michaels S. *The Social Organization of Sexuality: Sexual Practices in the United States*. Chicago, Ill: University of Chicago Press; 1994. Also see: Michael RT, Laumann EO, Kolata G, Gagnon JH. *Sex in America: A Definitive Survey*. Boston, Mass: Little, Brown & Co; 1994.
20. From: "Gloria Stewart, 75, Jimmy Stewart's wife of 44 years." *The Pittsburgh Post-Gazette*. February 8, 1994; Obituaries:C-8.
21. Baxter N, Coher R, McLeod R. The impact of gender on the choice of surgery as a career. *Am J Surg*. 1996;172:373-376.
22. Bolton-Maggs P, Van Someren V, Lefford F. The need for part-time work: a survey of doctors 10 years after graduation. *Br J Hosp Med*. 1988;39:413-418.
23. Redman S, Saltman D, Straton J, Young B, Paul C. Determinants of career choices among women and men medical students and interns. *Med Educ*. 1994;28:361-371.
24. Slomski AJ. Women in groups: barriers keep falling but frustrations persist. *Med Economics*. 1994; December12:39-59.
25. Moore EE. Presidential address: swimming with the sharks—without the family being eaten alive. *Surgery*. 1990;108:125-138.
26. Simpson LA, Grant L. Sources and magnitude of job stress among physicians. *J Behav Med*. 1991;14:27-42.
27. Novack DH, Suchman AL, Clark W, Epstein RM, Najberg E, Kaplan C. Calibrating the physician: personal awareness and effective patient care. *JAMA*. 1997;278:502-509.
28. Resident Forum. AMA-RPS instrumental in achieving new maternity leave policy. *JAMA*. 1991;265:1756.

Further Reading

For further information on the effect of divorce on children:

Spruijt E, de Goede MJ. Transitions in family structure and adolescent well-being. *Adolescence*. 1997;32:897-991.

Cherlin AJ, Chase-Lansdale L, McRae C. Effects of parental divorce on mental health through the life course. *Am Sociol Rev*. 1998;:239-249.

Zill N, Schoenborn CA. *Developmental, Learning, and Emotional Problems: Health of Our Nation's Children, United States, 1988*. Hyattsville, Md: National Center for Health Statistics; 1990. Advance Data from Vital and Health Statistics, No. 120.

McLanahan S, Sandefur G. *Growing Up With a Single Parent.* Cambridge, Mass: Harvard University Press; 1994.

For information on the call for greater attention to physician well-being:

Novack DH, Suchman A, Clark W, Epstein RM, Najberg E, Kaplan C. Calibrating the physiciaan: personal awareness and effective patient care. *JAMA.* 1997;278:502-509.

Index

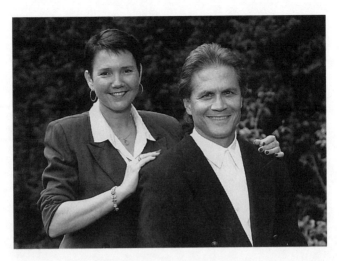

Wayne M. Sotile, Ph.D., and Mary O. Sotile, M.A. are co-directors of Sotile Psychological Associates, PLLC and Real Talk, Inc., in Winston-Salem, North Carolina, where Wayne also serves as Director of Psychological Services at the Wake Forest University Cardiac Rehabilitation Program. They have authored five books, including *Beat Stress Together: The BEST Way to a Passionate Marriage, a Healthy Family, and a Productive Life* (Wiley: 1999; Audio: 1999). The Sotiles' work on work/family balance and the management of interpersonal relationships in the medical workplace has been featured in the professional literature and in the international popular media, including national television. The Sotiles serve as consultants regarding interpersonal dynamics to numerous medical practices and hospitals. They are also among the most sought-after speakers and workshop leaders, having presented more than 1,000 keynotes to gatherings of medical professionals.